江苏大学英文教材基金资助出版

HISTOLOGY

组织学

卢小东
（Lu Xiaodong） 主编

江苏大学出版社
JIANGSU UNIVERSITY PRESS
镇 江

图书在版编目(CIP)数据

组织学＝Histology：英文/卢小东主编. —镇江：江苏大学出版社，2017.12
ISBN 978-7-5684-0734-2

Ⅰ.①组… Ⅱ.①卢… Ⅲ.①人体组织学－教材－英文 Ⅳ.①R329

中国版本图书馆 CIP 数据核字(2017)第 327014 号

组织学

HISTOLOGY

主　　编/卢小东
责任编辑/仲　蕙
出版发行/江苏大学出版社
地　　址/江苏省镇江市梦溪园巷 30 号(邮编：212003)
电　　话/0511-84446464(传真)
网　　址/http：//press.ujs.edu.cn
排　　版/镇江文苑制版印刷有限责任公司
印　　刷/虎彩印艺股份有限公司
开　　本/787 mm×1 092 mm　1/16
印　　张/10.5
字　　数/360 千字
版　　次/2017 年 12 月第 1 版　2017 年 12 月第 1 次印刷
书　　号/ISBN 978-7-5684-0734-2
定　　价/48.00 元

如有印装质量问题请与本社营销部联系(电话：0511-84440882)

PREFACE

Histology is the science of microscopic structures and functions of normal human beings. It provides the basic knowledge concerning how the human body is composed and how it functions at the levels of cell and tissue, which is the foundation for understanding the mechanisms of diseases. Histology, therefore, is usually a compulsory course in the curricula of undergraduate medical students. This is a concise textbook of histology, covering the histological aspects of tissues, organs and systems of almost the whole body. The book is aimed to aid undergraduate medical students to establish the principle conceptions of the structures and functions of human body after they have finished the study of the course, and readily to understand how the diseases occur and develop when they start to learn pathology.

I thank our team, including Dr. Chen Qian Dr. Wu Weijiang, Dr. Zhou Zhengrong and Dr. Yang Wenjing. With the collaborations of the team members, we gained rich experience in tutoring the international students, which is beneficial for me to write the book. I also thank those who provided the aids in publishing this book, including the sponsor Overseas Education College of Jiangsu University, the editor Ms. Zhong Hui, Mr. Qian Baoming for his help of processing the figures and Mr. Calvin Yee Fan Lee for his review and comments of the manuscript.

Dr. Lu Xiaodong

CONTENTS

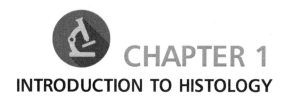

CHAPTER 1
INTRODUCTION TO HISTOLOGY

Histology is the branch of the anatomical sciences, focusing upon the normal microscopic structures of the human body as well as their related functions. Via studying histology, we will complete the knowledge of human body's structures from gross to microscopic; be able to understand how the different tissues function, which is the basis of physiology; and know the prelude of pathology for diseases are known only after the normal. The knowledge of histology which is the foundation of clinic sciences enables us to become a good doctor in the future.

Cells are the smallest structural and functional units in the body. Tissues are composed of groups of cells and the surrounding support media (extracellular matrix). Four primary tissue types are categorized into epithelial tissue, connective tissue, muscle tissue and nerve tissue. The cells within these categories of tissues may vary in structure and be specialized according to their function and location.

Microscope used in the study of histology is categorized into light microscope (LM) and electron microscope (EM). Microscopic structure is the structure seen with the aids of a microscope. LM structure is measured with the unit of micrometer(μm, 1000 μm =1 mm); and EM structure is measured with nanometer (μm,1000 nm =1 μm).

The resolution or resolving power of the LM is 0.2 μm. Resolution is the smallest distance between two points that can be observed separately.

1.1 Light Microscopy

HE-stained paraffin-embedded section is the routine method used in the study of histology. With this method, very thin slices of tissues, several micrometers thick, are prepared through which light can penetrate. To achieve sufficient contrast and colors in the tissues so that they may be visualized, dyes or specific chemicals are applied to the slices of tissues. Steps required in preparing tissues include fixation, dehydration and clearing, embedding, sectioning, mounting and staining the sections.

1.1.1 Fixation

Fixation is the treatment of the tissue with chemical agents that not only retard the alterations of the tissue subsequent after removal from the body, but also maintain its normal architecture. The most common fixative agent is formalin, which cross-links proteins, therefore maintaining a life-like image of the tissue.

1.1.2 Dehydration and clearing

Because a large fraction of the tissue is composed of water, a graded series of alcohol is used to remove the water. The process is called dehydration. The tissue is then treated with xylene, a chemical that is miscible both with alcohol and melted paraffin. This process is known as clearing because the tissue becomes transparent in xylene.

1.1.3 Embedding

Most body tissues are soft in life and only a little harder after they have been fixed in formaldehyde, so they are difficult to slice thinly enough for light microscopy examination. In order to prepare thin slices, tissue samples are impregnated with a substance which makes them solid. The usual embedding medium is paraffin. The tissue is placed in melted paraffin until it is completely infiltrated. The sample in the melted wax is then set and cooled; and a solid block of wax forms in which the tissue sample is embedded. The tissue is then ready for sectioning.

1.1.4 Sectioning

The blocks of tissue are sectioned using a microtome, a machine equipped with a blade and an arm that moves the tissue block in specific equal increments. For light microscopy, the thickness of each section is about $5 \sim 10$ μm, and each section or a series of sections is mounted on glass slides. Sectioning can also be performed on specimens frozen either in liquid nitrogen or on the rapid-freeze bar of a cryostat.

1.1.5 Staining

As most staining methods use dyes soluble in water, wax-embedded tissue sections have to be processed through the reverse of the sequence of solvents used to embed the tissues in order to remove the wax and return the tissue sample to an aqueous solution. The most commonly-used dyes are haematoxylin and eosin (H&E). Tissue components that stain readily with the basic dyes (e.g. haematoxylin) are called basophilic; those with an affinity for acid dyes (e.g. eosin) are termed acidophilic. Tissue components that do not readily stain with both basic and acid dyes are called neutrophilic.

In the figures of this book, the sections are the sections of paraffin-embedded and hematoxylin-eosin stained, if not specifically indicated. The low, middle and high magnification is respectively referred to the original magnification of 100, 200 and 400 times, respectively.

Certain dyes stain tissue components a different color from that of the dye solution. The color change in the dye is called metachromasia. Some tissue structures can be visualized with silver impregnation in which silver ions are deposited on tissues showing brown to black color, thus the structures are known as argyrophilic.

After staining, the section is again dehydrated so that the coverslip may be permanently affixed by the use of a suitable mounting medium.

1.2 Electronic Microscopy

Transmission electron microscopy uses much thinner sections compared with light microscopy and requires heavy metal precipitation techniques rather than water-soluble stains to stain tissues. In this method, beam of electrons instead of visible light and electromagnetic fields in place of glass lenses are used (Fig. 1-1). The resolution of the EM is about 0.2 nm. The same principles of a transmission electron microscope are involved as for the LM, with the following differences:

◆ Double fixation in glutaraldehyde and osmium tetroxide is employed.

◆ Ultrathin sections are cut from plastic embedded blocks.

◆ Heavy metal salts such as lead citrate or uranyl acetate are used for staining.

Unlike transmission electron microscopy, scanning electron microscopy is used to view the surface of a specimen. Using this technique, one can view a three dimensional image of the object. Usually, the object to be viewed is prepared in a special manner that permits a thin layer of heavy metal, such as gold or palladium, to be deposited on the specimen's surface.

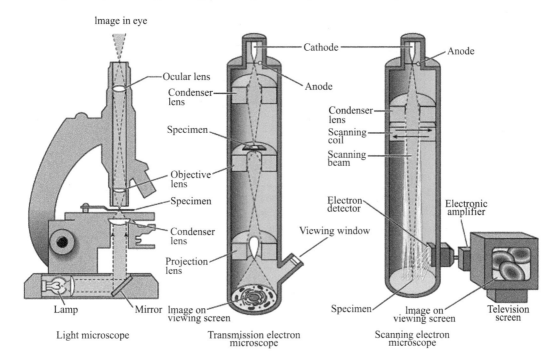

Fig. 1-1 Comparison of LM and EM

1.3 Histochemistry and Cytochemistry

The study of the chemical compositions of tissues and cells *in situ* by both microscopic and chemical analysis, i. e. , by chemical reactions producing insoluble colored compounds observed with the LM, or electron scattering of precipitates observed with the EM.

1.3.1 PAS reaction

PAS reaction is a method to detect polysaccharides, in which periodic acid oxidizes glycol groups in the glucose residues into aldehyde groups, which then react with Schiff reagent giving rise to an insoluble compound with a reddish purple color.

1.3.2 Immunocytochemistry

Immunocytochemistry is a very sensitive method for identification of a cell or tissue constituent *in situ* by means of a specific antigen-antibody reaction tagged by a visible label. The body produces specific proteins called antibodies, in response to invaded foreign proteins called antigens, and the antibodies then react with the antigens. An antibody can be linked to a fluorescent dye, horseradish peroxidase or colloidal gold so that the sites where immunological reactions occur can be localized.

1.4   Interpretation of Microscopic Sections

One of the most difficult skills needed in histology is to learn how to interpret what a two-dimensional section looks like in three dimensions. If one imagines a blood vessel as in Fig. 1-2 and then takes the indicated thin sections from that vessel, one can mentally reconstruct the correct three-dimensional image.

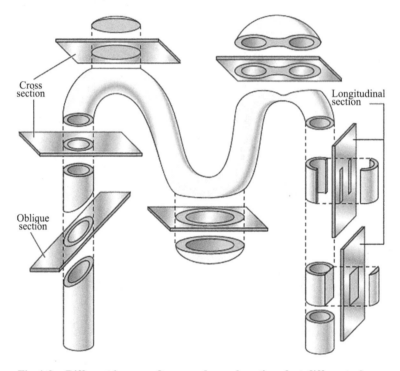

Fig. 1-2   Different images of a curved vessel sectioned at different planes

CHAPTER 2
EPITHELIUM

Epithelium is one of the four basic tissues, with wide distribution on the surface and many functions. It consists of continuous sheets of cells with very little extracellular substance. It covers body surfaces and also lines internal cavities. Epithelial cells are polarized, which means having the free surface, basal surface and lateral surfaces. Free surface is the apical surface free of the contact with any other cells; basal surface is in contact with an underlying basement membrane; and lateral surfaces are between adjacent cells. The epithelium has no blood vessels but rich in nerve terminals. Nutrients are diffused from the underlying connective tissue crossing basement membrane. Epithelia have numerous functions such as protection, synthesis, secretion, absorption and sensory reception.

Epithelium is categorized into two classes: covering and glandular. Covering epithelia cover body surfaces and line body cavities. It is classified according to the number of cell layers and the shape of the surface layer. Glandular epithelia have the function of secretion.

2.1 Covering Epithelia

2.1.1 Simple epithelia

Simple epithelium consists of one single layer of epithelial cells.

I. Simple squamous epithelium

Simple squamous epithelium consists of a single layer of flattened cells (Fig. 2-1). The nuclei are centrally-located and a bulge may be apparent in the region of the nucleus position. Simple squamous epithelia form the endothelial lining of blood and lymph vessels as well as the mesothelium of the pleural, pericardial, and peritoneal cavities. They also line pulmonary alveoli, compose the loop of Henle and the parietal layer of Bowman capsule in the kidney. The smooth surface facilitates the transport of gases and/ or other substances across the epithelium.

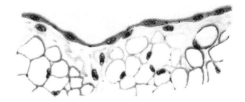

Fig. 2-1　Simple squamous epithelium

II. Simple cuboidal epithelium

Simple cuboidal epithelium is a single layer of cuboidal-shaped cells (Fig. 2-2). When viewed in a section cut perpendicular to the surface, the cells

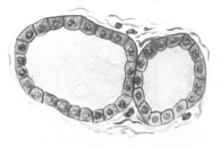

Fig. 2-2　Simple cuboidal epithelium

present a square profile with a centrally placed round nucleus. Simple cuboidal epithelia compose many kidney tubules and are found in thyroid. They function in protection, secretion and absorption.

III. Simple columnar epithelium

Simple columnar epithelium consists of one layer of cells that look like closely packed slender columns (Fig. 2-3). The ovoid nucleus is centrally or basally located. Simple columnar epithelium lines stomach, intestine, uterus, gallbladder, etc. Free surfaces of cells often bear microvilli, the thin fingerlike projections. When microvilli are closely packed, they form a striated border.

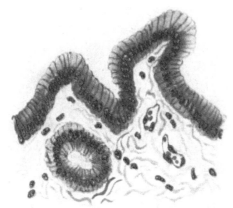

Fig. 2-3   Simple columnar epithelium

IV. Pseudostratified columnar epithelium

This type of epithelium is called "pseudostratified" because it appears as though it were composed of several layers but each cell actually has an attachment to the basement membrane. It appears multi-layered because some cells do not reach the surface (Fig. 2-4). This type of epithelium lines much of the respiratory tract. Some specialized epithelial cells in this "respiratory" epithelium produce mucus, which are unicellular glands, known as goblet cells; and others have cytoplasmic projections on their luminal surface known as cilia. Together, cilia and mucus entrap solid particles and the cilia can give rise to a powerful swaying, thus to compel the mucus towards the pharynx and expel it out via coughing.

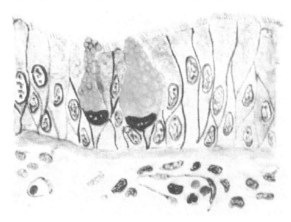

Fig. 2-4   Pseudostratified columnar epithelium

2.1.2 Stratified epithelia

Stratified epithelium consists of more than one single layer of epithelial cells.

Ⅰ. Stratified squamous epithelium

Stratified squamous epithelium is a type of multilayered epithelium that mainly protects against abrasion and dehydration (Fig. 2-5). It also prevents invasion of pathogens. It is subdivided into two types: keratinized and non-keratinized. In areas exposed to air and subject to abrasion, such as epidermis of skin, it is lined by keratinized stratified squamous epithelium, whose surface layer consists of dead cells lacking nuclei and containing the protein keratin. In other areas covered with fluid and with a moist surface (e. g. the oral cavity, esophagus, vagina, ect.), it is lined by non-keratinized stratified squamous epithelium, which has no keratinized layer.

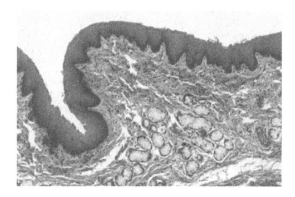 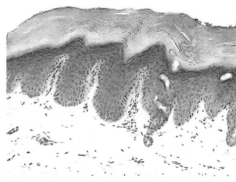

(a) Non-keratinized, of esophagus   (b) Keratinized, of skin

Fig. 2-5   Stratified squamous epithelium

The squamous surface cells are shed, especially when abrasion occurs, but they are replaced by deeper cells which become flattened as they move to the surface layer. Cells located at the base of the epithelium are the progenitor (stem) cells. Mitosis of these stem cells ensures that the layers of cells are constantly replaced as some new cells migrate to the surface. Importantly, some cells remain in the basal layer and continue to function as stem cells.

Ⅱ. Transitional epithelium

This type of epithelium is a highly specialized stratified epithelium present only in the urinary tract, e. g. the innermost of urinary bladder (Fig. 2-6). The appearance of transitional epithelium depends on the amount it is stretched. In an empty bladder, numerous epithelial cell layers are apparent. As the volume of urine in the bladder increases, the surface epithelial cells become flattened and the number of layers of cells is reduced.

The most superficial layer in contact with the lumen consists of relatively large, often binucleate cells. Their free surfaces are more convex in empty condition and they span several cells underneath, so they are called umbrella cells. Their apical cell membranes may show densely stained crust-like plaques in HE sections.

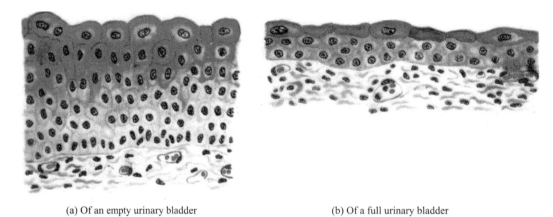

(a) Of an empty urinary bladder   (b) Of a full urinary bladder

Fig. 2-6　Transitional epithelium

2.2　Specializations of Epithelial Cells

The specialized structures on the surfaces of epithelial cells are present, and also can be seen between cells in other tissue. The specialized structures on respective surface will be discussed as following.

2.2.1　Specializations on free surface

I . Microvilli

Microvilli are the finger-like projections of the free surface membrane. In the microvilli microfilaments are found running longitudinally and extending into apical cytoplasm to insert in the terminal web. Clumps of microvilli may be visible as the striated border. Microvilli increase the surface area of absorptive cells in small intestine. (Fig. 2-7)

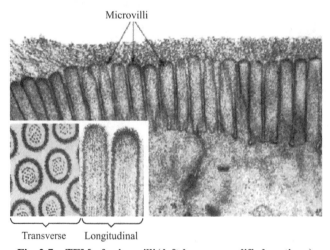

Fig. 2-7　TEM of microvilli(left lower, amplified sections)

II . Cilia

Cilia are slender projections from a cell surface. Internal structure is longitudinal "9 +2" microtubules, i. e. nine pairs of fused microtubules around the periphery and two central individual microtubules. Cilia beat in a wavelike fashion to sweep the epithelial surface clean. (Fig. 2-8)

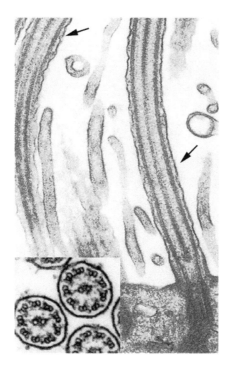

Fig. 2-8   TEM of cilia(arrows: longitudinal section; left lower: transverse section)

2.2.2   Specializations on lateral surface

I . Tight junction

Tight junction (or zonula occludens) is belt-shaped, encircling the apex of a columnar epithelial cell and sealing it to its neighbors. It is seen with the EM as the fusion of the outer leaflets of the cell membrane of adjacent cells in the form of discrete points (ridges). Tight junction functions in joining cells to form an impermeable barrier between the adjacent cells. (Fig. 2-9a)

II . Intermediate junction

Intermediate junction (or zonula adherens) is circumferential belt-like junction found just below a tight junction. It consists of an electron-dense plaque on the cytoplasmic faces of the adjacent cell membranes and a space between two plaques. The filaments of the terminal web in the apical cytoplasm are inserted into the dense plaques. Cells are connected tightly by the intermediate junctions between them. (Fig. 2-9b)

III. Desmosome

Desmosome (or macula adherens) is disc-shaped, very firm, and well-developed in the epidermis. A central line in the extracellular space is slightly widened. Transmembrane filaments span the cell membrane joining the plaque to the central line. Attachment plaques are dense materials deposited on inner surfaces of the adjacent cell membranes. The filaments in the cytoplasm are inserted into the plaques and then make a hairpin loop returning to the cytoplasm. (Fig. 2-9c)

IV. Gap Junction

Gap junction (or communicating junction) is the button-like junction between the two cells. Intermembranous protein particles (connexons) are tube-like and composed of six subunits. Two connexons in opposing membranes are in contact with a channel. Adjacent cells communicate small molecules and ions, and allow spread of electric impulses. (Fig. 2-9d)

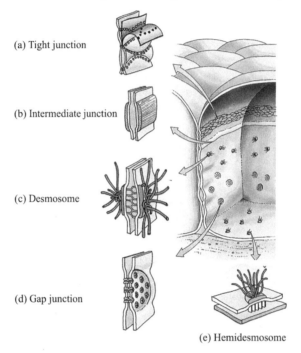

(a) Tight junction

(b) Intermediate junction

(c) Desmosome

(d) Gap junction

(e) Hemidesmosome

Fig. 2-9　Specializations on lateral surface

V. Junctional complex

Junctional complex means a close arrangement of several (two or more) cell junctions.

2.2.3　Specializations on basal surface

I. Basement membrane

Basement or basal membrane is a thin, sheet-like extracellular matrix, on which epithelial tissues rest. In EM, basement membrane is composed of basal lamina and reticular lamina. The basal lamina is generated by epithelial cells, containing the light-stained lamina lucida and darkly-stained lamina densa (basal lamina). The reticular lamina is located beneath the basal lamina, produced by the underlining connective tissue. The reticular lamina may be missing in some epithelia (Fig. 2-10). Basement membrane is not only a support for epithelia, but also a semi-permeable membrane through which the avascular epithelia get nutrients.

II. Plasma membrane infolding

The cell membrane of basal surface was invaginated into the cytoplasm, forming the plasma membrane infoldings. The infoldings are usually accompanied by longitudinally arranged mitochondria. These infoldings increase the basal surface area and enhance the passage of water and ions. They are well-developed in the renal tubules of the kidney. (Fig. 2-11)

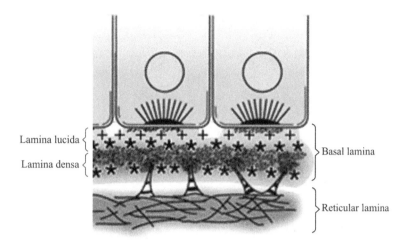

Lamina lucida
Lamina densa
Basal lamina
Reticular lamina

Fig. 2-10   Diagram of basement membrane

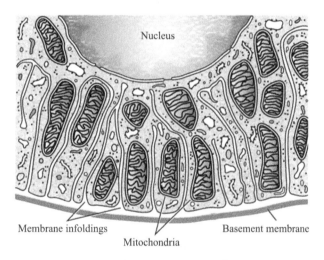

Nucleus

Membrane infoldings
Mitochondria
Basement membrane

Fig. 2-11   Plasma membrane infoldings

Ⅲ. Hemidesmosome

Hemidesmosome takes the shape of half of a desmosome, and strengthens the cell adhesion to the basement membrane. (Fig. 2-9e)

2.3 Glandular Epithelia

Glandular epithelia are derived from covering epithelia, which descend into connective tissue. Glandular epithelia make up glands, and the structures that give rise to secretions. Glands are classified into exocrine glands and endocrine glands. Exocrine glands retain their connection with the surface epithelia from which they originated, and release their secretions through ducts onto the surface or in the cavity. Endocrine glands are ductless, and their secretions are released into the connective tissue spaces and transported by the bloodstream (see chapter 13 and 14).

CHAPTER 3
CONNECTIVE TISSUE

Connective tissue is a type of primary tissue, characterized by relatively few cells embedded within a large amount of extracellular matrix (ECM), which is composed of fibers and amorphous ground substance. This tissue develops from the mesenchyme, and is widely distributed in the body. Connective tissue is divided into connective tissue proper and specialized connective tissue. Connective tissue proper includes loose connective tissue, dense connective tissue, adipose tissue and reticular tissue. Cartilage, bone and blood are specialized connective tissue. Connective tissue provides mechanical support and connection; extravascular transport of nutrients, wastes, gases, hormones, etc; repairing, healing and defense.

3.1 Loose Connective Tissue

Loose connective tissue is composed of a loose arrangement of fibers and dispersed cells embedded in abundant gel-like ground substance and extracellular fluid (tissue fluid). The major component is ground substance with a few cells and fibers, thus loose connective tissue is soft and flexible. (Fig. 3-1)

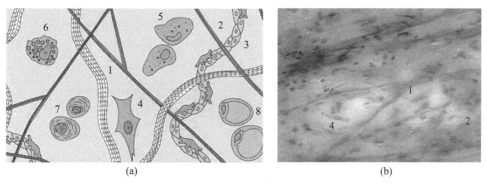

(a) (b)

1—Collagenous fiber; 2—Elastic fiber; 3—Capillary; 4—fibroblast;
5—Macrophage; 6—Mast cell; 7—Plasma cell; 8—Fat cell

Fig. 3-1　The diagram (a) and the mount (b) of loose connective tissue

3.1.1 Cells

I. Fibroblasts/Fibrocytes

Fibroblasts are the most numerous, responsible for secretion of fibers and ground substance. They are classified into two distinct morphologic and functional types: fibroblasts and fibrocytes.

Fibroblast is the young and active cell with an ovoid, large and pale-stained nucleus with prominent nucleolus and basophilic cytoplasm. EM reveals abundant RER and well-developed Golgi apparatus in the cytoplasm (Fig. 3-2). Fibroblasts secrete long, fiber-like protein molecules (e. g. collagen and elastin) and many of the other large molecules in the extracellular matrix. The mature and inactive cell (fibrocyte) is smaller with a dark, elongated nucleus. Fibroblasts are quiescent in the normal tissue. They are extremely active and fibrocytes may revert to fibroblast state in damaged tissue, undergoing mitosis and to synthesize new matrix for repair.

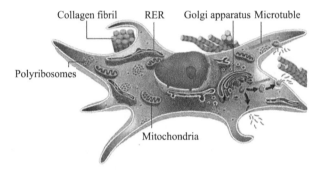

Fig. 3-2　Diagram of fibroblast

Ⅱ. Macrophages

Macrophage is oval or irregular in shape with an oval to round nucleus, and the acidophilic cytoplasm. They are characterized under the EM by ruffled surface and many lysosomes in the cytoplasm (Fig. 3-3). The macrophages are derived from blood monocytes. After entry into connective tissue, the monocytes enlarge and increase their lysosomes and phagocytic activity. The functions of these cells include: phagocytosis and digestion of microorganisms, damaged cells and foreign particles; capturing, processing and presenting antigens to lymphocytes triggering immune responses; secretion of a wide variety of substances such as lysozyme, interferon, interleukin, etc.

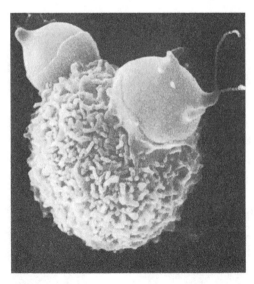

Fig. 3-3　SEM: a macrophage was phagocytosing two old red blood cells

III. Plasma cells

Plasma cells are scattered in loose connective tissue and especially in the lamina propria of the gastrointestinal tract, respiratory tract and in lymphatic organs. These cells are ovoid with an eccentric, cartwheel-like nucleus and basophilic cytoplasm, which contains rich RER and well-developed Golgi apparatus in the EM. Plasma cells synthesize and secrete immunoglobulin (antibody). (Fig. 3-4)

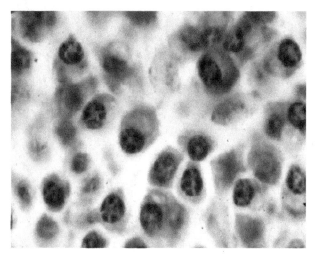

Fig. 3-4   Plasma cells

IV. Mast cells

Mast cells are often located near blood vessels, containing abundant and coarse basophilic granules, which are metachromatic. These cells respond to antigenic stimulus with a rapid release of histamine, heparin, leukotriene and other substances. When released from mast cells, these molecules modify the permeability of blood vessels as part of an inflammatory reaction. Degranulation is mediated through the binding of specific antigen to specific IgE, which is previously bound to specific IgE receptor on the mast cell membrane. (Fig. 3-5)

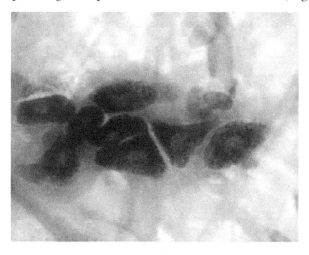

Fig. 3-5   Mast cells

Ⅴ. Fat cells

A fat cell (adipocyte) contains a single droplet of lipid, and looks like a signet ring in routine sections. These cells synthesize and store lipid. (Fig. 3-6)

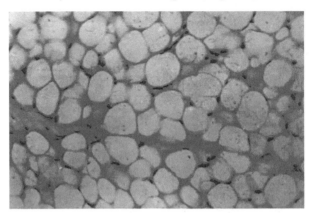

Fig. 3-6   Fat cells in the section

Ⅵ. Undifferentiated mesenchymal cells

These cells exist along small blood vessels, and can differentiate into fibroblasts.

Ⅶ. Leukocytes

Neutrophils and eosinophils enter connective tissue and live there for a short time and die. Lymphocytes enter the tissue and leave mostly through the lymphatic vessel and return to the blood circulation. During infections, inflammation and other pathologic conditions, leukocytes increase in number, and they are involved in defense.

3.1.2 Fibers

Fibers in connective tissue are classified into three types on the basis of their morphology and reactivity with histological stains: collagenous, elastic and reticular.

Ⅰ. Collagenous fibers

They are the most abundant type of fibers, white in fresh conditions. Fibers go singly or in bundles and branch. In LM, collagenous fiber appears as wavy bands, pink with HE stains (Fig. 3-1). In EM, it consists of bundles of fibrils, longitudinal section of which shows cross-bandings with axial periodicity of 64 nm. These fibers have great tensile strength, but inelastic. The chemical composition is collagen (type Ⅰ and type Ⅲ).

Ⅱ. Elastic fibers

They are yellow in fresh conditions and not readily seen in the LM unless special stains are used. In LM, the elastic fiber is slender, straight and branching. In EM, the fiber has central amorphous elastin and peripheral microfibrils. Elastic fibers impart resilience and elasticity of tissue. (Fig. 3-1)

Ⅲ. Reticular fibers

They are delicate fibers forming a fish-net for support of many individual cells (fat cells, smooth muscle cells, etc) and other structures (blood vessels, glands, nerve fibers, etc). These fibers are not seen in HE sections, but high affinity for silver stain, thus also known as argyrophilic fiber. (Fig. 3-7)

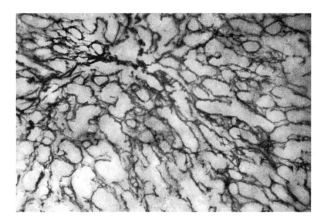

Fig. 3-7   Reticular fibers（silver-stained）

3.1.3   Ground substance

Ground substance is an amorphous gel-like material composed of glycosaminoglycans, proteoglycans, and glycoproteins. Tissue fluid is present in ground substance. Macromolecules in the ground substance act as a molecular sieve permitting nutrients, gases and metabolites to pass through and being a barrier to bacteria from spreading.

3.2   Other Connective Tissue Proper

3.2.1   Dense connective tissue

Dense connective tissue has great amount of fibers over cells and ground substance, classified into regular and irregular.

I. Dense regular connective tissue

In dense regular connective tissue, collagen fiber bundles are parallel and tightly packed. They are distributed in tendons, aponeuroses, ligaments and cornea. (Fig. 3-8)

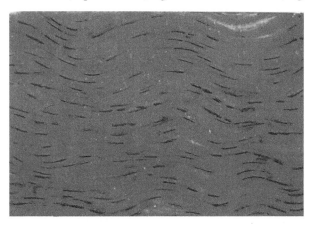

Fig. 3-8   Dense regular connective tissue

II. Dense irregular connective tissue

In dense irregular connective tissue, collagen fiber bundles are randomly interwoven into a network. They are distributed in dermis, capsules of various organs, perichondrium, etc.

3.2.2　Elastic tissue

Elastic tissue is composed of parallel elastic fibers and they are found in yellow ligaments and walls of large arteries.

3.2.3　Adipose tissue

Adipose tissue is made up of large aggregation of fat cells in loose connective tissue and found in hypodermis, mesenteries, perirenal region, etc. It serves as an energy storage, shock-absorber and insulating layer to conserve body heat.

3.2.4　Reticular tissue

Reticular tissue is composed of reticular cells and reticular fibers, and forms the architectural framework of lymphatic and hematopoietic tissues. Reticular cells are stellate with a large, pale nucleus and processes, which contact with those of neighboring cells to form a network.

CHAPTER 4
CARTILAGE AND BONE

Cartilage and bone are specialized forms of connective tissue. Together with other connective tissue and skeletal muscle they constitute the musculoskeletal system. Common features of bone and cartilage are that they contain connective tissue fibers and ground substance, forming an extracellular matrix which is relatively rigid compared with the rest of the body and is able to resist mechanical stress.

4.1 Cartilage

Cartilage is composed of cartilage matrix and cells (chondrocytes). Cartilage is categorized into three types according to the kind and amount of predominant fibers: hyaline cartilage, elastic cartilage and fibrocartilage.

4.1.1 Hyaline cartilage

Hyaline cartilage is the most abundant cartilage of the body. It is located in respiratory passages (from nose to bronchi), ventral ends of ribs and articular ends of bones in a joint. (Fig. 4-1)

I. Cartilage matrix

The semitranslucent blue-gray matrix of hyaline cartilage contains up to 40% of its dry weight in collagen. Its chemical composition is similar to that of connective tissue matrix, but

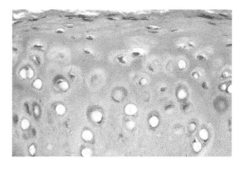

Fig. 4-1　Hyaline cartilage

chondroitin-SO_4 is main molecule, so the matrix is basophilic in HE sections. The delicate collagen fibrils which is made up of type II collagen, are dispersed in the matrix. Because the refractive index of the collagen fibrils and that of the ground substance are nearly the same, the matrix appears to be an amorphous mass with the light microscope. Blood vessels are absent in the matrix. The matrix has small cavities called lacunae occupied by cells. Matrix close to the lacuna is more intensely stained than the remaining and called territorial matrix.

II. Chondrocytes

The chondrocytes are located in the lacunae. Those chondrocytes near the periphery are flat ovoid, whereas those deeper in the cartilage are more rounded. Toward the center, cells are round and mature, arranged in groups. One group of the cells are derived from one single cell by mitosis of the cell, thus the group is called the isogenous group. EM of the chondrocyte demonstrates abundant RER and well-developed Golgi complex, responsible for synthesis and secretion of matrix.

III. Perichondrium

Dense connective tissue sheath around the cartilage forms the perichondrium. Outer fibrous layer is protective and inner layer is rich in blood vessels and cells.

IV. Growth of hyaline cartilage

Growth in hyaline cartilage occurs by two modes: interstitial growth and appositional growth.

i. Interstitial growth

Interstitial growth (growth from within) occurs mainly in the early stage of cartilage development. In interstitial growth, preexisting chondrocytes divide to increase the number of cells and amount of matrix from within.

ii. Appositional growth

Appositional growth occurs at the periphery of clusters of cartilage cells, adjacent to the perichondrium. Fibroblasts in the innermost part of the perichondrium are known as chondrogenic cells because they can become chondroblasts and secrete cartilage matrix. Most cartilage in the body grows by appositional growth.

4.1.2 Elastic cartilage

There are structural similarities between the elastic cartilage and hyaline cartilage. However, the matrix of elastic cartilage contains type II collagen fibers, but in addition, it has an abundance of elastin fibers which confer on the cartilage a degree of deformability and recoil. The elastin fibers are displayed using special stains. Elastic cartilage is present in epiglottis and the external ear. (Fig. 4-2)

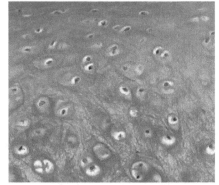

Fig. 4-2 Elastic cartilage

4.1.3 Fibrocartilage

Fibrocartilage is present in intervertebral disks, pubic symphysis and articular disks. The chondrocytes in fibrocartilage often appear oriented along the lines of stress on the cartilage, and there are intervening layers of collagen fibers (type I). Fibrocartilage provides resistance to mechanical forces. (Fig. 4-3)

4.2 Bone

Bone tissue is a kind of specialized connective tissue with calcified matrix, thus more rigid than cartilage, and provides support, movement, protection and a storage site for calcium.

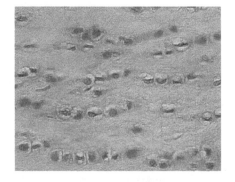

Fig. 4-3 Fibrocartilage

4.2.1 Bone matrix

The extracellular matrix of bone tissue is known as bone matrix. The components of bone matrix are organic part and inorganic part. Organic part is mostly collagen fibers (90%), and also ground substance (proteoglycans, osteocalcin, osteonectin, osteopontin). The inorganic part consists largely of calcium hydroxyapatite $[Ca_{10}(PO_4)_6(OH)_2]$. The hydroxyapatite is deposited alongside the collagen fibers and this produces the rigid hardness of bone, imparting resilience to bone.

4.2.2   Bone lamellae

Bone lamella is the basic structural form of bone matrix. Bone matrix is arranged in plywood-like layers with the fibrils parallel in one layer and rectangular between adjacent layers. The bone matrix layers are known as bone lamellae. Needles of hydroxyapatite lie alongside the collagen fibrils.

4.2.3   Bone cells

There are four types of cells present in the bone tissue: osteoprogenitor cells, osteoblasts, osteocytes and osteoclasts. (Fig. 4-4)

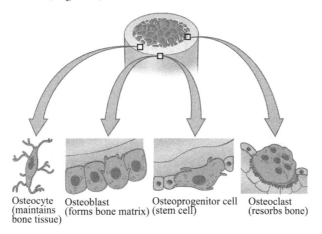

Osteocyte (maintains bone tissue)   Osteoblast (forms bone matrix)   Osteoprogenitor cell (stem cell)   Osteoclast (resorbs bone)

Fig. 4-4   Four types of cells present in the bone tissue

I. Osteoprogenitor cells

These cells are stem cells, located on the surface of the osseous tissue, and differentiate into osteoblasts when osteogenesis is active.

II. Osteoblasts

Osteoblasts are the cells developing from osteoprogenitor cells, located at the surface of bone tissue and responsible for producing the bone matrix. Osteoblasts are cuboidal cells with a large pale nucleus and basophilic cytoplasm. Abundant RER and Golgi in EM indicate active protein synthesis. Newly-formed, uncalcified organic matrix is called osteoid. Osteoid is soon calcified with calcium salt deposition initiated by matrix vesicles probably derived from osteoblasts.

III. Osteocytes

Osteoblasts are mature bone cells. Osteoblasts become trapped inside the calcified matrix and become osteocytes. They no longer produce osteoid and lose most of RER and basophilia, and become flattened. The cell bodies of these cells are located in the lacunae, and cytoplasmic processes are held in canaliculi. The cytoplasmic processes form gap junctions with adjacent osteocytes, providing for intercellular communication. Osteocytes with their processes are bathed in tissue fluid, which are from blood vessels in Haversian canals.

IV. Osteoclasts

Osteoclasts are bone resorptive cells, often found in depression on the bone surface involved in bone resorption. These cells are giant multinucleated cells, irregular in shape and acidophilic, formed by fusion of monocytes. The ruffled border (irregular microvilli) on the surface adjacent to bone and lysosomes in the cytoplasm are evidence of bone resorption. The lysosomal enzymes and organic acids are released into extracellular space to break down organic and mineral components of bone.

4.2.4　Bone structure

Most bones in the body contain compact (dense) and spongy (cancellous) bone. Compact bone is very dense compared with spongy bone. In a typical adult long bone, compact bone forms an outer collar along the shaft (diaphysis), whereas spongy bone constitutes the less dense interior. Spongy bone forms most of the ends of long bones (the epiphyses). The shaft of the long bone harbors bone marrow in the central cavity. (Fig. 4-5)

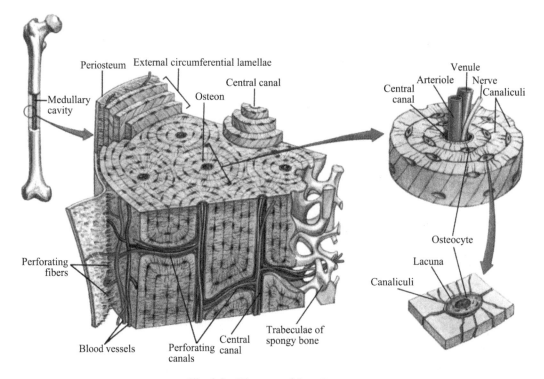

Fig. 4-5　Diagram of long bone

I . Compact bone

In compact bone, the bone lamellae are arranged in three patterns: circumferential lamellae, osteons and interstitial lamellae.

i . Circumferential lamellae

Circumferential lamellae are the parallel bone lamellae that surround the outer or inner circumferences of the diaphysis. The outer circumferential lamellae are just deep to the periosteum and the inner circumferential lamellae, completely encircle the marrow cavity. Trabeculae of spongy bone extend from the inner circumferential lamellae into the marrow cavity.

ii . Osteons

Osteons (or Haversian systems) are the structural units of compact bone. It contains several concentrically arranged lamellae and a central canal (Haversian canal) with connective tissue, blood vessels, and nerves. Between or within bone lamellae are living cells (osteocytes) in lacunae connected to one another by canaliculi, Volkmann's canals crossly perforate the circumferential lamellae and bring blood vessels into the Haversian canals, nourishing the compact bone. (Fig.4-5, Fig.4-6)

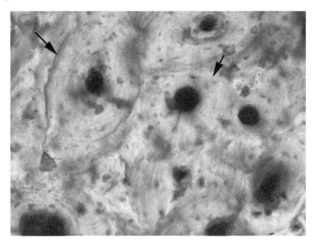

Fig.4-6   Bone ground (arrows: osteons)

iii . Interstitial lamellae

Interstitial lamellae are irregular and fill spaces between osteons, and derived from older osteons partially removed.

II . Spongy bone

Spongy bone is typically found at the ends of long bones, near to joints and within the interior of vertebrae. Spongy bone is highly vascular and frequently contains red bone marrow where haematopoiesis, the production of blood cells, occurs. The primary anatomical and functional unit of spongy bone is the trabecula.

III . Periosteum and endosteum

Periosteum is a layer of dense connective tissue covering the external surface of bone. Endosteum is a thin layer of bone lining cells on inner surface of bone. Osteoprogenitors are usually located beneath the periosteum or endosteum.

IV . Bone formation and growth

Bone formation and growth begin in embryonic stage and continue up to the age of 20 or so. After this time, ossification and bone growth stop but the components of matrix are gradually removed and/or replaced throughout life. In addition, at any stage, the shape of bones may be remodelled in response to various factors including dietary changes, strenuous exercise or physical damage. Bone formation and growth occur by two methods: intramembranous and endochondral ossification.

i . Intramembranous ossification

This type of bone formation and growth is associated only with flat bones. In regions where these bones develop, some fibroblast-like cells (osteoprogenitor cells) derived from mesoderm of the embryo differentiate into osteoblasts which then secrete osteoid. Growth occurs as osteoprogenitor cells differentiate and become osteoblasts which then produce bone matrix onto the existing matrix, i. e. by appositional growth.

ii . Endochondral ossification

The majority of bones in the skeletal system are formed by endochondral ossification. In this process a "model" of hyaline cartilage, comprising chondrocytes and cartilage matrix in the shape of the adult bone, develops first. The cartilage model grows and gradually bone matrix and bone cells replace the cartilage in the diaphysis. In growing long bones the diaphysis is separated from each epiphysis by an epiphyseal growth plate (EGP) of cartilage. This is the region where many bones grow in length.

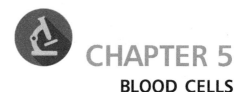

CHAPTER 5
BLOOD CELLS

Blood, the red, viscous, slightly alkaline fluid (pH, 7.4) is a kind of specialized connective tissue. The total volume of blood of an average adult is about 5 L, and it circulates throughout the body within the confines of the circulatory system. Blood is composed of formed elements (blood cells) and the extracellular matrix, known as plasma. The blood cells contain red blood cells (RBCs; erythrocytes), white blood cells (WBCs; leukocytes), and platelets. (Fig. 5-1)

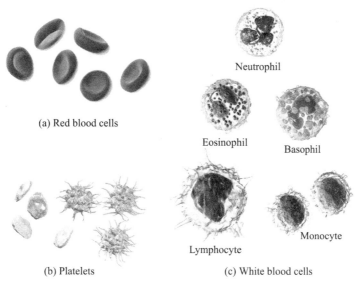

(a) Red blood cells

Neutrophil

Eosinophil

Basophil

(b) Platelets

Lymphocyte

Monocyte

(c) White blood cells

Fig. 5-1   Diagram of blood cells

As blood circulates throughout the body, it is an ideal vehicle for the transport of materials, which includes conveying nutrients from the gastrointestinal system to all of the cells of the body and subsequently delivering the waste products of these cells to specific organs for elimination. Metabolites of the cells, hormones and other signaling molecules, and gasses are also ferried by the bloodstream to their final destinations.

Blood cells are observed by blood smear, routinely stained with Wright's or Giemsa's stains. (Fig. 5-2)

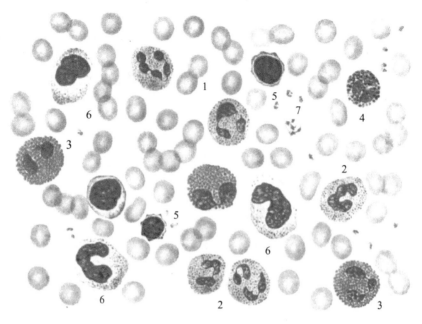

1—Red blood cells; 2—Neutrophils; 3—Eosinophils; 4—Basophil;

5—Lymphocytes; 6—Monocytes; 7—Platelets

Fig. 5-2   Blood smear (Wright's stain)

5.1   Blood Cells

5.1.1   Erythrocytes (red blood cells, RBCs)

The erythrocytes are the most numerous blood cells, about 5×10^{12} per liter blood. Mature erythrocytes are biconcave discs approximately 7.5 μm in diameter. In blood smears, erythrocytes usually appear rounded and have palely stained centers. The erythrocytes have no nucleus and no organelles. In the cytoplasm, it is filled with hemoglobin (Hb). Hb combines with and transports O_2 and CO_2 between the lungs and tissues. The unique shape of the erythrocyte provides larger surface area and shorter distance for gases to diffuse than if it were a sphere. Erythrocytes are very flexible, which enable themselves to change shape and pass through capillaries.

The cell membrane of the RBC has specific antigens and determines the blood group. The most notable of these are the A, B, and O antigens, which determine the four primary blood groups, A, B, AB, and O. People who lack either the A or B antigen, or both, have antibodies against the missing antigen in their blood (Fig. 5-3); if they undergo transfusion with blood containing the missing antigen, the donor erythrocytes are attacked by the recipient's serum antibodies and are eventually lysed.

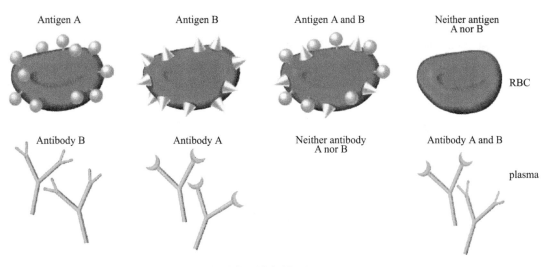

Antigen A　　　Antigen B　　　Antigen A and B　　Neither antigen
　　　　　　　　　　　　　　　　　　　　　　　　　A nor B

RBC

Antibody B　　　Antibody A　　Neither antibody　　Antibody A and B
　　　　　　　　　　　　　　　　　A nor B

plasma

Fig. 5-3　ABO blood group

The reticulocytes are immature RBCs with organelle remnants such as mitochondria and ribosome, visible as a mesh-like network with specific staining. They take up 0.5% ~1.5% of blood RBCs and are the indicator of hematopoietic capacity of the bone marrow.

Erythrocytes have a life span of approximately 120 days and after this time they are destroyed by cells in the liver, spleen and bone marrow.

5.1.2　Leukocytes (white blood cells, WBCs)

Leucocytes are referred to as white blood cells because of their whitish color in the zone between plasma and red blood cells after centrifugation of blood. Leukocytes are spherical and nucleated cells, with the number about $(4 \sim 10) \times 10^9$ per liter blood. Leukocytes are categorized into granulocytes and agranulocytes, depending upon presence or absence of the specific granules in the cytoplasm. Leucocytes with specific granules are granulocytes, which are subcategorized into neutrophils, eosinophils, and basophils. Leucocytes without specific granules are agranulocytes, which contains only non-specific granules. Non-specific granules are the granules that can be stained sky-blue by azure dyes, thus they are also known as azurophilic granules. In EM, the azurophilic granules are lysosome. Agranulocytes are subcategorized into monocytes and lymphocytes.

I. Neutrophils

Neutrophils are the most numerous leukocytes, about 60% ~70% of the total number of leucocytes. Neutrophils are 9 ~12 μm in diameter and have a multilobed nucleus, usually 2 ~5 lobes, increasing in number with the age of the cell. The lobes are connected by thin threads of chromatin. In their cytoplasm, two types of granules (azurophilic and neutrophilic) exist, both fine and stain weakly pink-purple. Azurophilic granules are lysosomes, larger but fewer than specific ones and contain peroxidase in addition to lysosomal enzymes. Neutrophilic granules contain lysozyme and phagocytes. Neutrophils phagocytose and kill bacteria. They accumulate in pus at the site of the infection. Increase in the number of neutrophils indicates acute bacterial infections.

II. Eosinophils

Eosinophils take up about 1% ~ 3% total leukocytes. The eosinophil has bilobed nucleus and its cytoplasm is usually filled with large granules stain bright pink. Eosinophils respond to antigen-antibody complexes and to parasites. They are able to phagocytose and digest antigen-antibody complexes and the remains of parasites. In addition, they release histaminase that destroys histamines and reduce the inflammatory processes. Eosinophils are present in increased numbers in blood and body tissues during allergic reaction and parasitic infections.

III. Basophils

Basophils are least encountered, about 0 ~ 1% total leukocytes. Basophilic granules are large, irregular in size and distribution, dark-purple, and obscure the nucleus. Granules contain histamine and heparin, like mast cells. Functions of these cells are not well understood, probably involved in allergic and inflammatory reactions.

IV. Lymphocytes

Lymphocytes make up 20% ~ 30% of the total number of leucocytes. Lymphocytes are also present in bone marrow, thymus, spleen and lymph nodes, and in lymphoid regions in other organs. They are 6 ~ 18 μm in diameter. Small lymphocytes are over 90% of the total, with round, indented nucleus containing dense chromatins. Thin rim of cytoplasm stains light-blue with a few azurophilic granules, lacking peroxidase.

Lymphocytes are classified into three classes: T-lymphocytes, B-lymphocytes, and NK cells depending upon the origin and surface antigen. T cells are involved in cell-mediated immunity in which T cells directly kill the target cells. B cells are involved in humoral immunity in which B cells give rise to plasma cells that secrete antibody against the antigen. NK cells migrate through body tissues and have the ability to detect and kill foreign cells.

V. Monocytes

Monocytes make up 3% ~ 8% of the total number of leucocytes. They are the largest cells in blood. The nucleuses of monocytes are more lightly stained than those of lymphocytes, with delicate chromatin. The nuclear shape varies from oval, kidney-like to horseshoe-like. Cytoplasm is basophilic and bluish-gray owing to many fine azurophilic granules, containing lysosomal enzymes and peroxidase. Monocytes migrate into tissues to become macrophages.

5.1.3 Thrombocytes (platelets)

Thrombocytes or platelets are about $(100 \sim 400) \times 10^9$ per liter blood, 2 ~ 4 μm in diameter. They are cytoplasmic fragments of megakaryocytes, a large cell type present in bone marrow. The cell has no nucleus and is biconvex disc in SEM; irregular-shaped in clusters or singly in LM. Platelets are released into blood vessels in bone marrow and they then circulate around the body. Platelets are essential for blood clotting and help control haemorrhage. They release vasoconstrictor (5-HT); adhere and aggregate to form platelet thrombus, and promote blood clotting to seal breaks of blood vessels.

5.2 Bone Marrow

Bone marrow occupies spaces within bones. Red blood cells, white blood cells and platelets develop in bone marrow in a process known as haematopoiesis. Within bone marrow blood flows in endothelium-lined blood vessels and a reticular meshwork surrounding the vessels is packed with developing blood cells. Macrophages are associated with the meshwork and they are involved in destroying aged red blood cells. Megakaryocytes are also in the meshwork and they shed fragments of their cytoplasm, as platelets, into adjacent blood vessels. The appearance of bone marrow in sections reveals few details of the structure of the developing blood cells and smears of bone marrow are examined for detailed studies. Megakaryocytes, however, can be identified readily in sectioned material by their large size and multilobed nucleus.

5.3   Haematopoiesis

All blood cells arise from one type of stem cell in bone marrow which resembles a small lymphocyte and is described as being pluripotent. These stem cells undergo successive rounds of mitosis and replace themselves and produce cells which are able to differentiate into different types of cells with restricted stem cell ability. After several cycles of mitotic activity, the potential to develop into several types of blood cell is restricted and unipotent stem cells develop.

Hematopoietic stem cells possess capacity of self-replication, strong proliferation and differentiation into multiple hematopoietic progenitor cells. Hematopoietic progenitor cells are unipotential or bipotential generate precursor cells, which in turn produce various mature blood cells.

Unipotent stem cells are committed to produce one type of blood cell and replace themselves. Unipotent stem cells are categorized by the type of blood cell they produce. The stages in the formation of erythrocytes, eosinophils, basophils, neutrophils, monocytes, T lymphocytes, B lymphocytes, NK cells and megakaryocytes from stem cells are shown in Fig. 5-4.

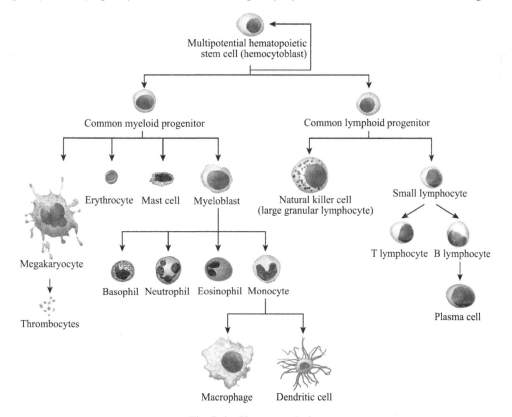

Fig. 5-4   Haematopoiesis

The rate of production of new blood cells in the bone marrow normally equals the rate at which each cell type dies, from less than a week to 120 days. Most blood cells leave bone marrow when they are mature by entering blood in vessels in bone marrow. Some cells, such as neutrophils, usually stay in the bone marrow for a few days after they mature and they act as a reservoir of cells that can rapidly enter the circulation and migrate to sites of infection.

The following Tab. 5-1 shows the morphologic criteria of blood cell development from immature to mature

Tab. 5-1   Morphologic criteria of blood cell development

Items	Morphologic alteration
Cell size	Larger→smaller (except megakaryocytes)
Nucleus size	Larger→smaller (disappears in RBCs)
Nucleus shape	Round→indented→lobed (granulocytes)
Chromatin	Delicate network→coarse condensed
Nucleolus	Several→not identified
Cytoplasm	Scanty, basophilic → plenty, acidophilic (agranulocytes still basophilic)
Specific components such as hemoglobin and specific granules	No→appear→increase
Nucleus/cytoplasm ratio	Larger→smaller
Division ability	Own→no (except lymphocytes)

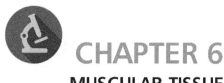

CHAPTER 6
MUSCULAR TISSUE

Muscular tissue is composed of muscle cells (muscle fibers) with connective tissue between them. Muscle fibers are elongated and highly differentiated cells, containing myofilaments and able to contract. The cell membrane is known as sarcolemma, the cytoplasm as sarcoplasm and the smooth endoplasmic reticulum (SER), as sarcoplasmic reticulum (SR). The connective tissue provides support of muscle fibers and brings in blood vessels and nerves.

Muscular tissue is divided into three types: skeletal, cardiac, and smooth muscle. The first two are striated due to a regularly repeated arrangement of striation in the longitudinal section of the muscle fibers. The smooth muscle is non-striated, due to the absence of the striations.

6.1 Skeletal Muscle

Skeletal muscle is composed of long, cylindrical, multinucleated cells that perform voluntary contraction. It is attached to bone via tendons, and associated with the skeleton, thus to provide movement of the body.

The connective tissue surrounding muscle cells consists of three covering layers. Each muscle cell is covered by and bound to, the fine connective tissue known as the endomysium. Several muscle cells are held together as bundles by the connective tissue coat known as the perimysium. The connective tissue layer covering entire

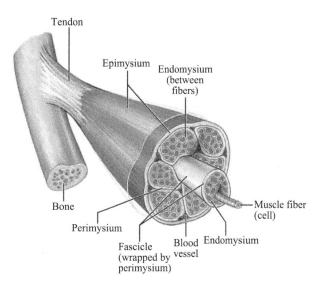

Fig. 6-1 Organization of skeletal muscle

muscle is known as the epimysium; and this layer is also known as deep fascia. (Fig. 6-1)

6.1.1 LM structures of the skeletal muscle fibers

Muscle fibers are long, cylindrical cells. They are multinucleated cells and the nuclei are elongated and lie beneath the sarcolemma. (Fig. 6-2)

In longitudinal section (along the length of the cells) of the skeletal muscle, display the cross striations, i. e. muscle fibers have alternating dark bands (or anisotropic bands, A bands) and light bands (or isotropicbands, I bands). The transverse section (cross the length of the cells) of skeletal muscle demonstrates the sarcoplasm of each muscle fiber eosinophilic stained and the punctuate appearance are the sections of bundles of myofibrils, which occupy much of the sarcoplasm of each cell. Numerous blood capillaries in the connective tissue layers around muscle cells are usually shown.

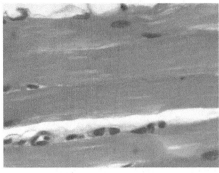 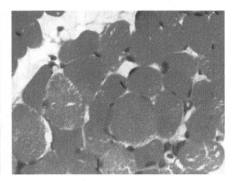

        (a) Longitudinal section   (b) Transverse section

Fig. 6-2　Sections of skeletal muscle

6.1.2　Ultrastructures of the skeletal muscle fibers

I. Myofibrils

The organelles myofibrils in the sarcoplasm are the basic structure for contraction. They are long, cylindrical structures arranged parallel each other in the muscle fibers. Taking one myofibril to study, the myofibril display A band and I band alternatively arranged. Z line is a dark line bisecting each I band. The shortest contractile unit of a myofibril is sarcomere, which is a segment of one myofibril between two consecutive Z lines. H band is light area in middle of A band. M line is present in middle of H band (Fig. 6-3).

Myofibrils are composed of myofilaments parallel to one another. The two types of filaments of myofilaments are thick filaments and thin filaments. (Fig. 6-3, Fig. 6-4)

i. Thick filaments

Thick filaments (or myosin filaments) occupy the A band. They are made up of myosin molecules.

◆ Myosin: Myosin molecules having a globular head and a rod. When assembling, the rods overlap and the heads direct toward either of the ends forming cross bridges. The head has ATPase, which is activated when the head binds the actin, the component of the thin filament.

ii. Thin filaments

Thin filaments are parallel to thick filaments. One end of a thin filament is inserted into and attached to the Z line, which is a web-like set of threads. The other end is free and extends into the A band. Thin filaments are composed of three types of protein: actin, tropomyosin and troponin.

◆ Actin: The monomers of actin is globular actin (G actin), which polymerize in the same head-to-tail orientation to form the two-strand helix, the F-actin. Each G actin has an active site that can bind to the head of a myosin molecule.

◆ Tropomyosin: The thin filament also has tropomyosin. Pencil-shaped tropomyosin molecules polymerize to form the slender double-stranded tropomyosin that occupies the shallow grooves of the double-stranded actin helix. The tropomyosin blocks the active sites of the thin filaments when the muscle is relaxed.

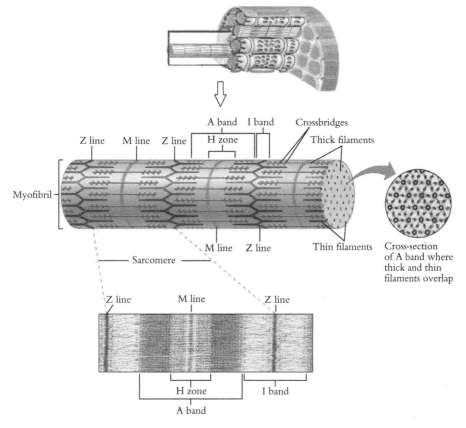

Fig. 6-3   **Thick filaments and thin filaments in a sarcomere**

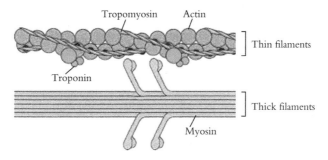

Fig. 6-4   **Molecular components of thick and thin filaments**

◆ Troponin: Troponin molecule is composed of three globular polypeptides: TnT, TnC, and TnI. The TnT subunit binds the entire troponin molecule to tropomyosin; TnC has a great affinity for calcium; and TnI binds to actin, preventing the interaction between actin and myosin. Binding of calcium by TnC induces a conformational shift in tropomyosin, exposing the previously blocked active sites on the actin filament so that myosin heads can bind to the active site on the actin molecule.

II. Transverse tubules (T tubules)

T tubules are formed by sarcolemma invagination into the sarcoplasm at the junction level between A and I bands. A complex anastomosing T tubules is formed encircling every myofibril at A-I junctions of each sarcomere. T tubules are responsible for rapid conduction of impulses to the interior of the muscle fiber. (Fig. 6-5)

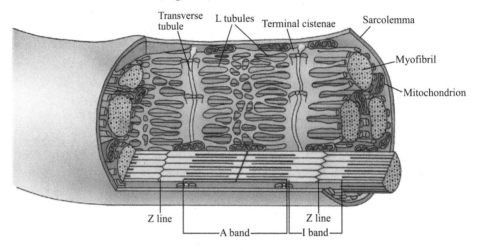

Fig. 6-5   T tubules and L tubules

III. Longitudinal tubules (L tubules)

Longitudinal tubules (L tubules), also known as sarcoplasmic reticulum (SR), consist of a branching network of smooth endoplasmic reticulum encircling each myofibril between two adjacent T tubules. At the ends of SR, L tubules are dilated and fused to form terminal cisternae, which are closely apposed to the T tubule. Each T tubule lies between the two terminal cisternae of the SR forming a triad. The role of SR is to store Ca^{2+} and regulate concentration of Ca^{2+} within the sarcoplasm.

Sarcoplasm of skeletal muscle fiber also has abundant mitochondria and glycogen granules. The mechanism of contraction relies upon "sliding filament hypothesis". When myofibril contracts, I band and sarcomere become shortened, H band disappears, and A band remains constant in length. The reason for the above suggests that thin filaments slide over thick filaments and insert further into the A band. Ca^{2+} and ATP play important roles in muscle contraction.

6.2   Cardiac Muscle

Cardiac muscle is found only in the heart with more connective tissue and capillaries between cardiac muscle fibers.

6.2.1   LM structure of cardiac muscle fibers

Cardiac muscle fibers are short column in shape and branched, each with a centrally placed nucleus. The muscle fibers show cross striations and myofibrils though the striations and myofibrils are less distinct. Cells link to one another end to end by intercalated discs. The intercalated discs are dark and thick striations, seen in the transverse section of cardiac muscle. (Fig. 6-6)

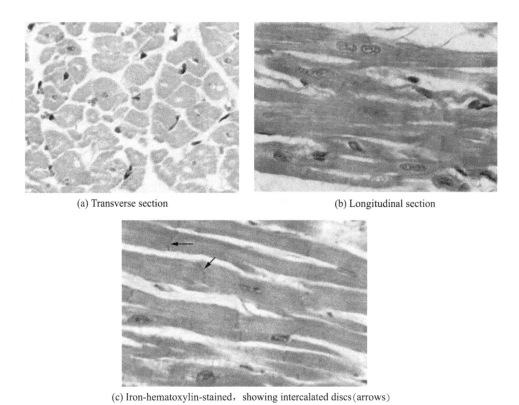

(a) Transverse section   (b) Longitudinal section

(c) Iron-hematoxylin-stained, showing intercalated discs(arrows)

Fig. 6-6   Sections of cardiac muscle

6.2.2   Ultrastructures of the cardiac muscle fibers

Compared with skeletal muscle fibers, T tubules of cardiac muscle fibers are thicker and at the level of Z lines. The sarcoplasmic reticulum is not well developed and longitudinal tubules expand into small terminal cisternae. T tubule often makes contact with the small terminal cisternae on one side to form a diad. Triads are not commonly found. Muscle cells have more sarcoplasm with more abundant mitochondria and glycogen to meet more energy demands. Intercalated discs are the specialized cell junctions at Z lines. Transverse portion has desmosomes and intermediate junctions to enhance intercellular junction. Longitudinal portion has gap junctions providing electrical continuity with adjacent cells, thus to maintain synchronous contraction of the muscle fibers. (Fig. 6-7)

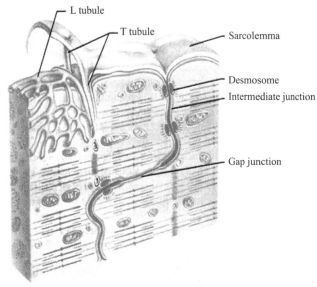

Fig. 6-7   Diagram of intercalated disc

6.3 Smooth Muscle

Smooth muscle is distributed in blood vessels and hollow viscera, usually arranged in layers. The muscle fibers are spindle in shape, with an elongated, centrally located nucleus (Fig. 6-8). The fibers have no striations, but containing thick filaments surrounded by thin filaments, the latter attached to dense bodies and patches.

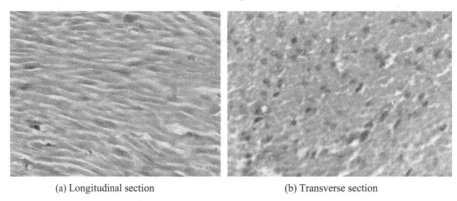

(a) Longitudinal section　　　　　　　　(b) Transverse section

Fig. 6-8　Sections of smooth muscle

Sarcolemma invaginates forming caveolae. Dense patches and dense bodies are located, respectively, beneath sarcolemma and in sarcoplasm, and connected by intermediate filaments (as cytoskeleton).

Adjacent cells are linked by gap junctions, so that contraction spreads from one cell to neighbors.

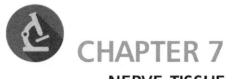

CHAPTER 7
NERVE TISSUE

Nerve tissue comprises neurons (nerve cells) and neuroglial cells. Neurons are responsible for the receptive, integrative, and motor functions of the nervous system. Neuroglial cells are responsible for supporting, protecting, and assisting neurons in neural transmission.

Nervous tissue makes up nervous system. The central nervous system consists of the brain and the spinal cord; and the peripheral nervous system comprises ganglia, nerves and nerve endings.

7.1 Neurons

Although the shape and size of neurons are variable, they all consist of two parts, the cell body (also known as perikaryon) and processes. The cell body of the neuron contains a large nucleus and perinuclear cytoplasm. The processes arise from the perikaryon and are of two forms, dendrites and axons. (Fig. 7-1)

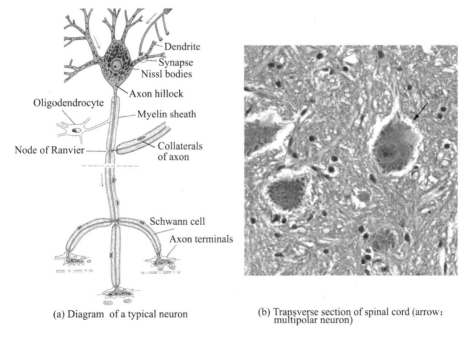

(a) Diagram of a typical neuron

(b) Transverse section of spinal cord (arrow: multipolar neuron)

Fig. 7-1 Structure of neuron

7.1.1 Cell body

The cell body is the metabolic, tropic and integral center of the neuron. The nucleus, located in the center of the cell body, is large, usually spherical. It contains finely dispersed chromatin and distinct nucleolus, indicative of intense synthetic activity.

The cytoplasm in the cell bodies often appears basophilic granules in HE-stained section, which are referred to as Nissl bodies; and in EM, they are clusters of RER and free ribosomes, indicating the active protein synthesis in the cytoplasm. Some of these proteins provide the structural tubules and filaments in axons and dendrites. Others are enzymes involved in producing molecules which aid the transmission of signals.

Neurofibrils are thin threads in the cell bodies and the processes of a neuron, visualized with silver staining in LM. They consist of neurofilaments and microtubules in bundles and therefore serve as cytoskeleton, and are involved in transportation of substances.

The organelles like Golgi complex, mitochondria and SER are also present in perikaryon. Moreover, melanin granules and lipofuscins, the yellowish brown pigment granules are seen in perikaryon.

7.1.2 Processes

The processes of neurons are two types: dendrites and axons.

I. Dendrites

The dendrites are the extensions of the cell body, thus contain similar organelles to perikarya, especially Nissl bodies. Dendrites usually are short and thick, and tapered as they branch and rebranch like a tree. Spines located on the surfaces of some dendrites permit them to form synapses with other neurons. One neuron has one or more dendrites. The main function of the dendrites is to receive information from other neurons and conduct it to the parent cell body.

II. Axons

Axons, usually long and thin with uniform diameter, do not branch profusely, but may have collaterals. An axon arises from a conical region called the axon hillock that derives from the perikaryon or occasionally from the stem of a major dendrite. The axon and axon hillock are devoid of Nissl bodies. One neuron has only one axon. The ends in several terminal branches of axons are called axon terminals or buttons, which contain vesicles with neurotransmitters in them. Axons conduct impulses away from one neuron to other neurons or to effector cells such as muscle or gland cells.

7.1.3 Ganglia and nuclei

Ganglia are the collections of neuronal cell bodies located outside the CNS. The equivalent aggregations of neuronal cell bodies in the CNS are known as nuclei. In addition to neuronal cell bodies, ganglia also contain supporting cells (satellite cells) and parts of the cytoplasmic processes (axons and dendrites) of neurons.

7.1.4 Classification of neurons

Neurons are classified into the groups according to the several criteria.

According to the number of processes, the neurons are divided into:

◆ Pseudounipolar neurons: The pseudounipolar neuron has one single process, which is soon divided into two in T-shape. This type of neurons are found in the spinal ganglion.

◆ Bipolar neurons: The bipolar neuron has one axon and one dendrite, present in cochlear and vestibular ganglia, retina, olfactory (receptor), etc.

◆ Multipolar neurons: The multipolar neuron has one axon and two or more dendrites. Majority of neurons are multipolar. (Fig. 7-2)

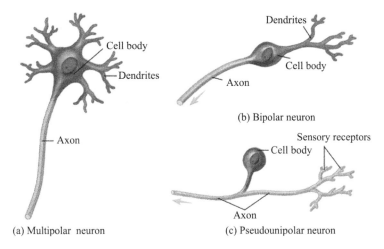

Fig. 7-2   Classification of neurons

According to the function, the neurons are divided into:

◆ Sensory or afferent neurons: They receive sensory stimuli from environment and from within the body, and conduct impulses to the central nervous system.

◆ Motor or efferent neurons: They conduct impulses to effector organs.

◆ Interneurons: they connect other neurons to form complex functional circuits, accounting for 99% of neurons in the body.

According to the neurotransmitters released, the neurons are divided into:

◆ Cholinergic neurons: They release acetylcholine from axon terminals.

◆ Aminergic neurons: They release catecholamines and other amines such as 5-hydroxytryptamine (5-HT).

◆ Peptidergic neurons: They release polypeptide neurotransmitters such as substance P.

7.1.5 Synapses

The synapse is the junction between two neurons or between a neuron and an effector cell, specialized for the transmission of impulses between the cells. There are two major types of synapses: chemical and electrical. The first uses a chemical mediator called neurotransmitter to transmit impulses from one cell to the next in one direction; the electrical synapse is gap junction, which permits direct flow of electrical current between two neurons.

Ⅰ. **Structure of chemical synapses**

The chemical synapses are composed of presynaptic elements, synaptic cleft and postsynaptic elements. (Fig. 7-3)

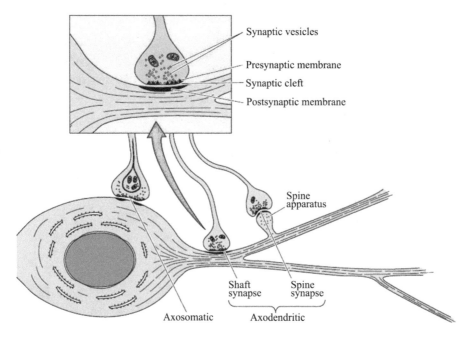

Synaptic vesicles

Presynaptic membrane

Synaptic cleft

Postsynaptic membrane

Spine apparatus

Shaft synapse

Spine synapse

Axosomatic

Axodendritic

Fig. 7-3　Structure of chemical synapses

i . Presynaptic elements

The presynaptic elements are usually formed by axon terminals which contain a population of synaptic vesicles. In EM, the vesicles are clear or dense. Clear vesicles contain acetylcholine (ACh) and dense core vesicles contain aminergic neurotransmitters or polypeptides. Presynaptic membrane is thickened and densely stained in EM.

ii . Synaptic cleft

The synaptic cleft is the extracellular space between presynaptic and postsynaptic membranes.

iii. Postsynaptic elements

The postsynaptic elements are usually dendrites (or spines) or cell bodies. The postsynaptic membrane is also thickened and possesses specific receptors to the neurotransmitter released from presynaptic element.

II . Classification of chemical synapses

Various types of synaptic contacts between neurons have been observed, as the following shows: **axodendritic synapse** (between an axon and a dendrite); **axosomatic synapse** (between an axon and a cell body); **axoaxonic synapse** (between two axons); **dendrodendritic synapse** (between two dendrites).

7.2　Neuroglia

Neuroglia are more than neurons by 5 ~ 10 times, and also have processes, but not conduct impulses. Only their nuclei can be seen with HE stains. Silver staining can demonstrate their processes and cytoplasm.

7.2.1　Neuroglia in the CNS

Four types of neuroglia present in the CNS: astrocytes, oligodendrocytes, microglia and ependymal cells. (Fig. 7-4)

I. Astrocytes

Astrocytes are the most numerous and the largest neuroglia, with an oval, pale staining nucleus and many processes. They are categorized into protoplasmic astrocytes and fibrous astrocytes. Protoplasmic astrocytes are stellate-shaped cells with abundant cytoplasm and many short branching processes. Fibrous astrocytes have long and unbranched processes. Astrocytes support and separate neurons, regulate neural activity, secrete neurotrophic factors, involved in repairing of the neurons. They participate in the forming of blood-brain barrier, which consists of tight junctions between endothelial cells of the capillaries, continuous basement membrane around endothelia and vascular feet of processes of astrocytes around capillaries.

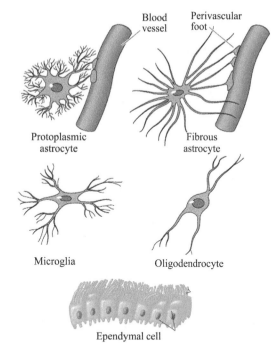

Fig. 7-4　Neuroglia in the CNS

II. Oligodendrocytes

Oligodendrocytes resemble astrocytes but are smaller. These neuroglial cells contain fewer processes with sparse branching and a round, dark-staining nucleus. They form myelin sheath around axons in the CNS.

III. Microglia

Microglia (or microglial cells) exhibit scant cytoplasm and irregular short processes. These cells function as phagocytes in clearing debris and damaged structures in the CNS. Microglia also protect the nervous system from microorganisms and tumor formation. They are derived from monocytes.

IV. Ependymal cells

Ependymal cells are low columnar to cuboidal epithelial cells, lining ventricles of the brain and the central canal of the spinal cord.

7.2.2　Neuroglia in the PNS

There are two types of neuroglia in the PNS: Schwann cells and satellite cells. (Fig. 7-5)

I. Schwann cells

Schwann cells (or neurolemmal cells) are flattened cells whose

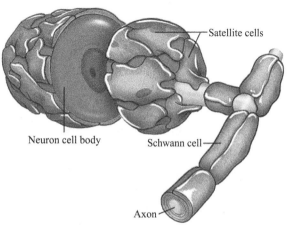

Fig. 7-5　Neuroglia in the PNS

cytoplasm contains a flattened nucleus. They envelop axons, forming either myelinated or unmyelinated coverings over the axons. They can guide nerve regeneration.

II. Satellite cells

Satellite cells (or capsular cells) are flattened cells, forming a kind of capsule around nerve cell bodies in the peripheral ganglia.

7.3 Nerve Fibers and Nerves

The long processes of neurons (usually axons), known as nerve fibers, are parallel one another. Each nerve is a cordlike structure containing bundles of axons and provides a common pathway for the electrochemical nerve impulses transmission. Within a nerve, each axon is surrounded by a layer of connective tissue called the endoneurium. The axons are bundled together into groups called fascicles, and each fascicle is wrapped in a layer of connective tissue called the perineurium. Finally, the entire nerve is wrapped in a layer of connective tissue called the epineurium. (Fig. 7-6)

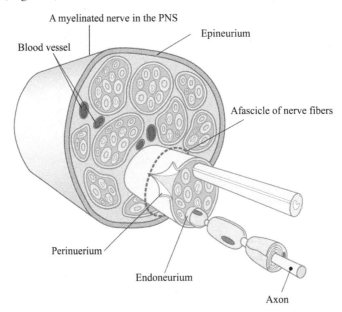

Fig. 7-6 Organization of myelinated nerve

There are two types of nerve fibers: myelinated and unmyelinated.

I. Myelinated nerves

Axons that have myelin wrapped around them are referred to as myelinated nerves. In the PNS, Schwann cells are the myelin-forming cells, whereas in the CNS oligodendrocytes are.

i. Myelinated nerves in the PNS

In the PNS, shown in EM, myelin is the plasmalemma of the Schwann cell organized into a sheath that is wrapped several times around the axon. Along its length the nerve fiber is segmented by the region devoid of myelin sheath and with bare portion of the axon, known as the nodes of Ranvier. The segment between two consecutive nodes of Ranvier is called an internode. The myelin sheath, arised from Schwann cell plasmalemma winding around the axon many times, contains lipids and proteins. In EM it shows a series of concentrically arranged lamellae, while in LM it is like a spongy structure because the lipids are dissolved out. The neurolemma is the outermost layer of cytoplasm, cell membrane and basal lamina of Schwann cells. (Fig. 7-7)

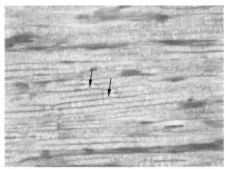 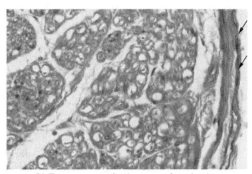

(a) Longitudinal section(arrows:nodes of Ranvier)   (b) Transverse section(arrows:epineurium)

Fig. 7-7   Section of myelinated nerve in the PNS

The myelin enhance the speed of conduction of impulse along them, i. e. impulses jumping from node to node, because myelin sheath serves as an insulator. The thicker axon has the thicker myelin sheath and the longer internode, and in turn has greater conduction velocity.

The myelin sheath shows cone-shaped clefts called clefts or incisures of Schmidt-Lanterman. These clefts, shown in EM, are the cytoplasm of Schwann cell trapped within the lamellae of myelin.

ii . Myelinated nerves in the CNS

In the CNS, the myelinated nerve fibers are similar as in the PNS. The flattened processes of oligodendrocytes are involved in the formation of myelinated nerves. No neurolemma and no incisures of Schmidt-Lanterman present in the CNS. (Fig. 7-8)

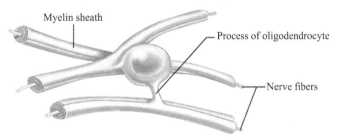

Fig. 7-8   Myelinated nerve fiber in the CNS

II . Unmyelinated nerve fibers

In the PNS, unmyelinated nerve fibers are axons engulfed by neighboring Schwann cells, with no myelin sheath and no nodes of Ranvier. In the CNS, unmyelinated nerve fibers run free among the other neural and glial processes.

III. Nerve endings

Nerve endings are classified into sensory and motor nerve endings.

i . Sensory nerve endings

Sensory nerve endings comprise free and encapsulated nerve endings.

A. Free nerve endings　Free nerve endings are the branches of naked nerve fibers. They are responsible for heat, cold, and pain. They are abundant in epidermis, cornea, etc.

B. Encapsulated nerve endings　Encapsulated nerve endings are the following:

◆ Tactile corpuscles: They are oval bodies with flattened cells, connective tissue capsule and nerve terminals. They are touch receptors and found in dermal papillae. (Fig. 7-9)

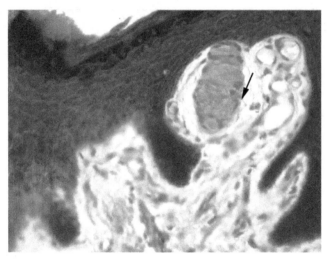

Fig. 7-9　Section of skin showing tactile corpuscle (arrow)

◆ Lamellar corpuscles: They are composed of concentric lamellae of flattened cells and internal cylinder with the naked axon inserted in it. They are distributed in subcutaneous tissue, mesentery and ligament. They perceive pressure and vibration. (Fig. 7-10)

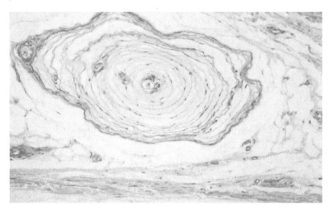

Fig. 7-10　Section of skin showing lamellar corpuscle

◆ Muscular spindles: They are spindle-like structure, distributed in skeletal muscle. They are responsible for the sense of the relative position and movement of the body. (Fig. 7-11)

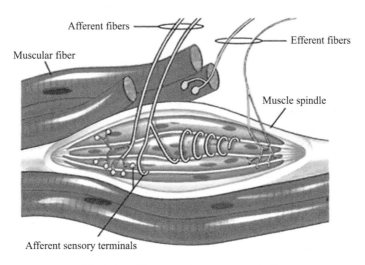

Fig. 7-11   Diagram of muscular spindle

ii . Motor nerve endings

Motor nerve endings include somatic and visceral. Somatic motor nerve endings are also known as motor ending plates. In LM, the ends of motor nerve fibers ramify with each terminal dilating as a plate-like mass and touching a muscle fiber. In EM, synapses with presynaptic elements contains acetylcholine and postsynaptic membrane (sarcolemma) contains the receptors for acetylcholine. A motor nerve fiber innervates many muscle fibers comprising a motor unit, whereas a muscle fiber is innervated by only one axon branch. (Fig. 7-12)

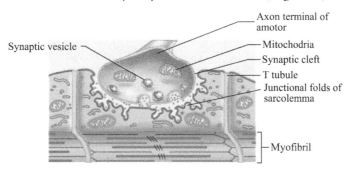

Fig. 7-12   Diagram of motor nerve ending

CHAPTER 8
SKIN

Skin, the largest organ, covers the whole surface of the body and is continuous at entry and exit points of the body with the mucous membranes lining the nose, mouth and anus, and the reproductive and urinary openings. The skin has roles in protection against microbes, physical and chemical damage and ultraviolet radiation; it also prevents excess water loss. Skin plays an important role in regulating body temperature by the ability of sweat glands to secrete sweat. In addition, the amount of blood flowing in vessels in the skin varies and this helps in regulating heat loss and thus body temperature too. Skin also has roles as a sense organ detecting stimuli through specific sensory nerve receptors. In addition, cells in the surface of skin exposed to sunlight are involved in the production of vitamin D.

The skin consists of two layers: the superficial epidermis and the deeper dermis consisting mainly of connective tissue. The dermis is superficial to the hypodermis and the latter is not considered to be part of the skin. The hypodermis is composed mainly of connective tissue, which may contain large numbers of adipose cells; the hypodermis is also known as superficial fascia or subcutaneous tissue. (Fig. 8-1)

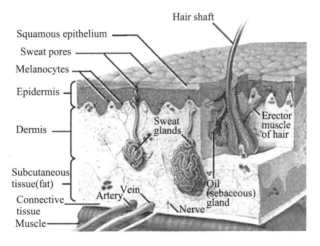

Fig. 8-1 Structure of skin

8.1 Epidermis

The epidermis is a kind of stratified squamous keratinized epithelium, and may be divided into five layers, though all layers are present only in thick skin, such as on the palms of the hand and soles of the feet.

8.1.1 Keratinocytes

Keratinocytes is composed of the following layers of epidermis. (Fig. 8-2)

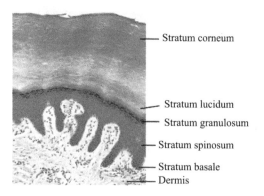

Fig. 8-2　Layers of epidermis

I. Stratum corneum

This is the most superficial layer and consists of the protein keratin. In thick skin the keratin is in numerous layers; there is less keratin in thin skin. Keratin is a filamentous protein produced by keratinocytes in deeper layers of the epidermis. It confers toughness and protection on the epidermis and helps to prevent water loss. Some keratin-forming cells in deeper layers produce lipids and this increases the ability of skin to resist water absorption. The surface of the stratum corneum is constantly being shed, particularly if it is subjected to abrasion. Importantly, the stratum corneum is constantly being added to as cells in the deeper layers move towards the surface.

II. Stratum lucidum

This is a thin layer, adjacent to the stratum corneum. The cells are packed with keratin and do not possess nuclei or organelles. They lose their cell membrane and become the basal layer of the stratum corneum. The change is rapid and the layer is seen only in the thickest skin.

III. Stratum granulosum

This layer is characterized by the presence of cytoplasmic granules of keratohyalin. Other cytoplasmic granules contain lipids and these are released into extracellular spaces and confer waterproofing of the epidermis. Upper cells in this stratum die and then become part of the stratum lucidum.

IV. Stratum spinosum

The thickest layer of the epidermis, the stratum spinosum, is composed of several layers of polyhedral to flattened cells. In cytoplasm, numerous bundles of intermediate (keratin) filaments are present, as well as coarse basophilic granules called keratohyalin granules, which have no limiting membrane. Another type of granules, known as lamellated granules contain lipid contents which can be discharged into intercellular spaces. The basally located keratinocytes in the stratum spinosum are mitotically active. The cells have numerous processes that give this layer a prickly appearance. Desmosomes are usually found between cells in this layer.

V. Stratum basale

This is the deepest layer of the epidermis and consists of a layer of cuboidal epithelial cells. The basal cells are attached to the basement membrane of the epidermis, which is adjacent to the dermis. The cells in this layer undergo mitosis and are the stem cells of the epidermis. Some offspring cells remain in this layer, undergo further mitotic activity, and thus continue as stem cells. Other offspring cells begin to produce keratin filaments and migrate towards the upper layer; this initially replaces the keratinocytes in the stratum spinosum. Over a period of about 30 days, keratinocytes produced by mitosis in the stratum basale migrate towards the surface of skin, die and the keratin they have formed is shed.

8.1.2 Non-keratinized cells

Within the epidermis there are various cell types in addition to keratinocytes. (Fig. 8-3)

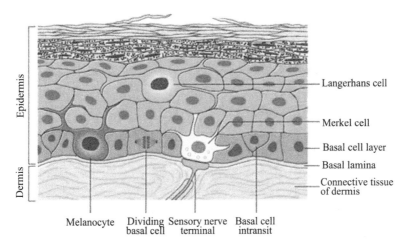

Fig. 8-3   A variety of cells in epidermis

I. Merkel cells

These cells are scattered throughout the stratum basale and are thought to act as mechanoreceptors.

II. Langerhans cells

These cells are derived from bone marrow cells and they have an immunological function. They are mainly located in the stratum spinosum.

III. Melanocytes

These cells produce pigment and are present in the stratum basale between the mitotically active cells. Melanin is responsible for the color of skin. The type and amount of pigment present is affected by the gene and the amount of exposure to ultraviolet light. Sunlight stimulates the synthesis and spread of melanin. Melanocytes have long cytoplasmic processes in which the melanin granules are present. They also pass melanin to keratinocytes. The melanin is often located in the cytoplasm of keratinocytes between the nucleus and the surface of the skin; there, it helps protect DNA from damage by ultraviolet light.

8.2 Dermis

Dermis consists largely of connective tissue fibers and cells. The dermis is divided into two layers, the papillary and the reticular layer.

I. Papillary layer

This is the most superficial layer and it interdigitates with the epidermis through a series of dermal ridges and papillae. In this way, the attachment of the epidermis and the dermis is strengthened. The papillary layer is characterized by loose connective tissue, rich in blood vessels that supply oxygen and nutrients to nearby epidermal cells and are involved in temperature regulation. Some sensory nerve endings are present in the papillary region of the dermis.

II. Reticular layer

The reticular layer is deep to the papillary layer and connects the skin to the underlying hypodermis. Dense irregular connective tissue containing many collagen fibers is predominant in the reticular layer.

8.3 Appendages of Skin

Appendages of skin comprise sweat gland, sebaceous gland, hair, arrector pilli muscle and nails (Fig. 8-4).

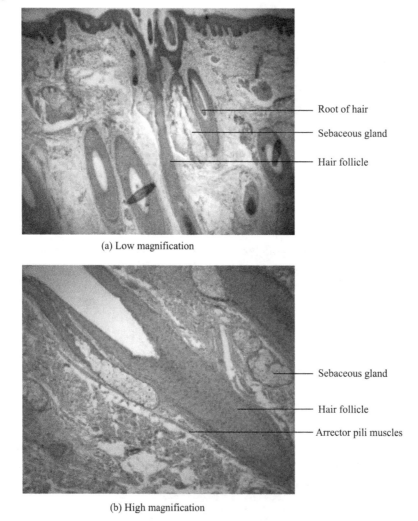

(a) Low magnification

(b) High magnification

Fig. 8-4 Section of the scalp

8.3.1 Sweat glands

Sweat glands of the skin include merocrine sweat glands and apocrine sweat glands sebaceous glands,

I. Merocrine sweat glands

They are present in skin all over the body and they are simple, coiled tubular glands. The secretory cells are located deep in the dermis, and even in the underlying hypodermis. An epithelial lined duct drains each gland and it passes to the superficial layer of the epidermis (stratum corneum). The duct is replaced by a spiral channel through the stratum corneum and opens at a pore on the surface of the skin. Merocrine sweat glands are innervated by sympathetic nerves and may be stimulated to secrete under conditions of stress.

II. Apocrine sweat glands

This type of sweat gland is present in the axilla, around nipples and in the anal region. The glands are larger than merocrine sweat glands, and they are located more deeply in the dermis and underlying hypodermis. Unlike merocrine glands, apocrine sweat glands do not secrete onto the surface of the skin; instead, they secrete around developing hairs in hair follicles. Secretion by apocrine sweat glands is influenced by sex hormones, and, after bacterial action, their secretions have a characteristic odor.

8.3.2 Sebaceous glands

Sebaceous glands secrete an oily substance known as sebum, which maintains the suppleness of the skin. Except for the palms of the hands, soles of the feet, and sides of the feet inferior to the hairline, sebaceous glands are found throughout the body. These glands are most abundant on the face, scalp, and forehead. Sebum is antimicrobial and assists in preventing watery fluids from entering or leaving skin. The activity of sebaceous glands is influenced by sex hormones and their activity increases substantially after puberty. The ducts of the sebaceous glands open into the follicular canal, where they discharge their secretory product to coat the hair shaft and, eventually, coat the skin surface.

8.3.3 Hair

Hair is formed largely of a compact, dense form of keratin. Each hair is produced in a structure known as a hair follicle. Hairs are widespread over the body surface though absent from the palms, soles, parts of the genitalia, tips of fingers and toes, and lips. Hairs are of two types: vellus hairs, which are the short, fine, soft hairs on the skin, and terminal hairs, which are the long hairs such as on the scalp. Hair follicles develop as cylindrical invaginations of the epidermis. Straight hair grows from straight follicles, and spiraling follicles give rise to curly hairs.

Hair follicles are surrounded by connective tissue. During the growing phase of a hair, the base of its follicle is expanded into a bulbous portion. An inner sheath, formed by cells produced in the hair bulb, extends only part way along the follicle. It is the innermost cells within the inner sheath which undergo keratinization and form the hair shaft. Each hair bulb is invaginated by a dermal papilla of connective tissue containing blood vessels which are essential for hair growth.

8.3.4 Arrector pili muscles

Arrector pili muscles are smooth muscle cells extending from midshaft of the hair follicle to the papillary layer of the dermis. Sympathetic nerves stimulate contraction of these smooth muscle cells and this causes hairs to "stand on end". Sympathetic nerves also supply sweat glands and the smooth muscle cells in the walls of blood vessels in the skin.

8.3.5 Nails

Nails are modifications of the stratum corneum of the epidermis on the dorsal aspect of terminal phalanges of fingers and toes. The nail plate is composed of multiple layers of squamous-shaped, keratinized cells that are firmly held together. These cells contain hard keratin and do not desquamate. The undersurface of both exposed and concealed parts of the nail plate is the nail bed. It consists of stratum basale of the epidermis and underlying dense dermis.

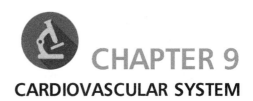

CHAPTER 9
CARDIOVASCULAR SYSTEM

The cardiovascular system is composed of the heart, a muscular organ that pumps the blood into two separated circuits: the pulmonary circuit, which carries blood to and from the lungs, and the systemic circuit, which distributes blood to and from all of the organs and tissues of the rest of the body. The components of these circuits are capillaries, arteries and veins.

9.1 Capillaries

Capillaries are the thin-walled vessels with the smallest diameter, where gases, nutrients, metabolic wastes, hormones, and signaling substances are interchanged or passed between the blood and the tissues of the body to sustain normal metabolic activities.

Capillaries arise from the terminal ends of arterioles. By branching and anastomosing, capillaries form capillary beds or capillary networks between the arterioles and the venules. These smallest blood vessels usually have a luminal diameter of $5 \sim 10 \mu m$, which is barely large enough for blood cells to squeeze along them.

Each capillary consists of an endothelium, an underlying basal lamina, and a few randomly scattered pericytes covered by a loose network of collagen and reticular fibers. Three types that vary in ultrastructure and permeability exist in the body: continuous, fenestrated, and sinusoidal. Their morphologic features are adapted to functional demands of specific organs and tissues. (Fig. 9-1)

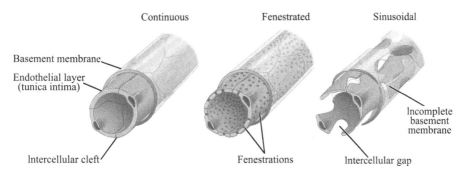

Fig. 9-1 Types of capillaries

9.1.1 Continuous capillaries

Continuous capillaries, the most common type, are found in all muscle tissues and in areas with a blood-tissue barrier. Continuous capillaries have uninterrupted endothelium. Their reduced permeability restricts indiscriminate passage of material from capillary lumen to surrounding tissues. Usually, desmosomes, and gap junctions link endothelial cells in these capillaries. Lipids and lipid-soluble molecules, including gases, diffuse freely across the endothelium, but larger water-soluble molecules are moved across the cells by pinocytosis. The pinocytotic vesicles engage in bidirectional pinocytosis by pinching off from endothelial surface membranes, moving across the cytoplasm, and discharging contents on the opposite surface.

An overlying basal lamina encloses the endothelium and surrounds occasional pericytes. Pericytes are mesenchymally derived pleuripotential stem cells and can differentiate into endothelial cells, in response to injury or stimulation by growth factors.

9.1.2　Fenestrated capillaries

Fenestrated capillaries are highly permeable, so they occur in areas engaged in active transport, e. g. the lamina propria of the intestines, glomeruli of the renal corpuscles, and some endocrine organs. Their endothelial cells are quite thin and held together by tight junctions and gap junctions, usually resting on a thin basal lamina. Pericytes are less numerous than in continuous capillaries. A unique feature is the presence of fenestrae, which are the round, small and transcellular pores in endothelial cells. A thin diaphragm usually closes each fenestra.

9.1.3　Sinusoidal capillaries

Sinusoidal capillaries (or sinusoid) have relatively wide and irregular lumens. They are found in bone marrow, spleen, liver, adenohypophysis, and adrenal cortex. The endothelial cells are separated by wide gaps through which fluid, large molecules, and blood cells may pass. At certain sites, such as sinusoids of liver and spleen, fixed macrophages are present and closely associated with sinusoidal endothelial cells. A basal lamina is either absent or incomplete.

9.2　General Structures of Blood Vessels

Except the very tiny blood vessels, three layers of tissue, or tunics, make up the wall of the typical blood vessel. They are from inner to outer: tunica intima, tunica media, and tunica adventitia. (Fig. 9-2)

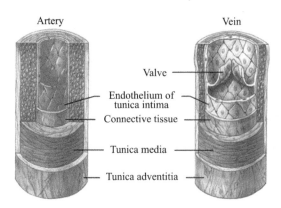

Fig. 9-2　Layers of blood vessels

Ⅰ. Tunica intima

The tunica intima is the innermost layer, composed of three sub-layers, as the following:
- ◆ Endothelial cells: a single layer of flattened, squamous endothelial cells, lining the lumen of the vessel.

◆ Subendothelial layer: the underlying subendothelial connective tissue.

◆ Internal elastic lamina: the thin band of elastic fibers that is well developed in medium-sized arteries.

II. Tunica media

The tunica media is composed mostly of smooth muscle cells and the connective tissue. In general, arteries closer to the heart have more elastin in this layer, and form numerous sheets of elastin. Arteries further from the heart have more smooth muscle than elastin in this layer. Generally veins have fewer smooth muscle cells in this layer than arteries.

III. Tunica adventitia

Tunica adventitia is composed mainly of fibroelastic connective tissue whose fibers are arranged longitudinally. Adjacent to the outer layer of the tunica media in some arteries, there is another band of elastic fibers, the external elastic lamina.

9.3   Arteries

Arteries are a series of vessels that transport blood away from the heart. Generally, arteries have thicker walls and are smaller in diameter than the corresponding veins. Moreover, in histological sections, arteries are round and usually have no blood in their lumen, whereas veins are irregular and frequently contain blood.

Arteries are classified into three major types based on their relative size. From largest to smallest, they are large (or elastic, conducting) arteries, medium-sized (or muscular, or distributing) arteries and arterioles.

9.3.1   Large arteries

Large arteries, e. g. aorta and pulmonary artery, are closest to the heart and conduct blood from the heart to muscular arteries. (Fig. 9-3)

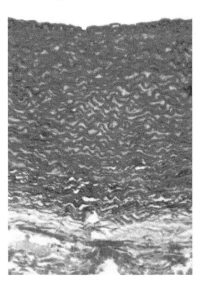

Fig. 9-3   Section of the large arteries

I. Tunica intima

The tunica intima is lined internally by an endothelium with its basal lamina. A deeper subendothelial layer of connective tissue consists mostly of collagen and elastic fibers embedded in ground substance, plus scattered fibroblasts and occasional smooth muscle cells. Underneath is a border of an internal elastic lamina, which is often difficult to discern as it merges imperceptibly with elastic laminae of the tunica media.

II. Tunica media

The tunica media in the wall of elastic vessels is the most prominent of three layers. It has abundant elastic fibers organized as multiple, concentric, fenestrated laminae, interspersed with scattered smooth muscle cells as well as some collagen. The number and thickness of elastic laminae vary with age: for example, in newborn aortas have about 25 concentric laminae, adult aortas, $50 \sim 75$.

III. Tunica adventitia

The tunica adventitia of these arteries consists of loose irregular connective tissue with a predominance of longitudinally oriented collagen fibers and scattered fibroblasts. In most elastic arteries, the adventitia contains small nutritive blood vessels (known as the vasa vasorum) and lymphatic capillaries. This microvasculature extends into the outermost part of the tunica media.

9.3.2 Medium-sized arteries

Medium-sized arteries are muscular arteries, for their predominant smooth muscle components. They distribute the blood from large arteries into organs. They vary greatly in size and can change their size markedly in response to functional demands. As muscular arteries become smaller, the number of elastic fibers and layers of smooth muscle gradually decrease.

Relative to the sizes of lumens, these arteries have thick walls. Their three layers are distinct, as the following: (Fig. 9-4)

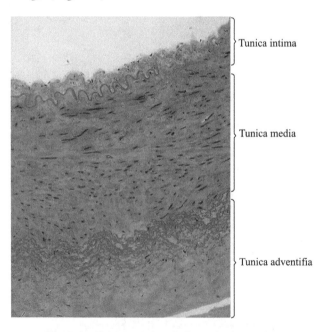

Tunica intima

Tunica media

Tunica adventifia

Fig. 9-4   Section of the medium-sized arteries

I. Tunica intima

The tunica intima in the muscular arteries is thinner than that in the elastic arteries, but the subendothelial layer contains a few smooth muscle cells; also, in contrast with that of elastic arteries, the internal elastic lamina of the muscular arteries is prominent and displays an undulating surface to which the endothelium conforms.

II. Tunica media

The identifying characteristic of medium-sized arteries is a relatively thick tunica media. This tunic is composed mostly of layers of circular smooth muscle cells, and may has as many as 40 layers. The number of muscle cell layers decreases as the diameter of the artery diminishes.

III. Tunica adventitia

The tunica adventitia of the muscular arteries consists of elastic fibers, collagen fibers and ground substance, produced by fibroblasts in the adventitia. Adjacent to the tunica media, an external elastic lamina is demonstrated as several layers of thin elastic fibers. The collagen and elastic fibers are oriented longitudinally and blend into the surrounding connective tissues. Located at the outer regions of the adventitia are vasa vasorum and unmyelinated nerve endings.

9.3.3 Arterioles

When the distributing arteries enter into the organs, they change into the arterioles. They share a pattern of layers in their walls similar to that of distributing arteries. However, they have only one to three layers of smooth muscle in the tunica media. The smooth muscle cells are arranged concentrically in the walls of arterioles and so their contraction and relaxation alters the diameter of their lumen. This contraction varies the amount of muscle tone and thus regulates blood flow into capillary beds. (Fig. 9-5)

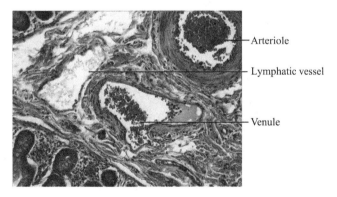

Fig. 9-5 Section of small intestine showing the arteriole, the venule and the lymph vessel

9.4 Veins

Veins are low-pressure blood vessels compared with arteries, and they return blood to the heart. In general, compared with arteries, there is much less smooth muscle and elastin and more collagen in the walls of veins. Furthermore, the ratio of luminal diameter to wall thickness is greater in veins than in adjacent arteries.

Veins may be grouped into small veins, medium veins and large veins. The smallest veins, venules, collect capillaries. In medium-sized veins, valves are present that prevent the back flow of blood. Valves are flap-like structures which have an endothelial covering and a fibrous core of connective tissue. The flaps project towards the heart; thus, if blood flow to the heart stops, the blood cannot pass backwards because the valve flaps are forced together and close the lumen. Valves are particularly important where there is a need to counteract the force of gravity such as in the limbs.

Interestingly, the superficial veins in the lower limbs in humans have a well developed component of smooth muscle in their walls which, by maintaining muscle tone, is thought to assist in preventing excess distension of the veins. The largest veins close to the heart do not have valves aiding unidirectional flow. Venous return from large veins below the heart is aided by pressure changes that occur in the thorax during inspiration and gravity aids venous return from the vessels above the heart.

9.5　Heart

The heart is a four-chambered pump of the cardiovascular system. The wall of the heart is divided into three layers from inner to outer: the endocardium, the myocardium and the epicardium. (Fig. 9-6, Fig. 9-7)

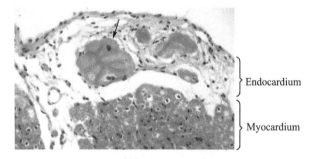

Fig. 9-6　Section of the heart showing the endocardium and the myocardium(arrow: Purkinje fibers)

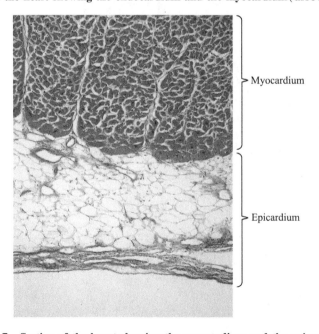

Fig. 9-7　Section of the heart showing the myocardium and the epicardium

9.5.1 Endocardium

The endocardium contains three sub-layers, from inner to outer as following:

Ⅰ. Endothelium

It is one layer of endothelial cells, which are the simple squamous epithelium.

Ⅱ. Subendothelial layer

This layer is beneath the endothelium, consisting of connective tissue with collagen fibers, elastic fibers, and scattered smooth muscle cells.

Ⅲ. Subendocardial layer

Deep in the endocardium is a subendocardial layer. It consists of loose connective tissue that contains small blood vessels, nerves, and Purkinje fibers from the conduction system of the heart.

9.5.2 Myocardium

The myocardium consists of interlacing bundles of cardiac muscle cells. The muscle fibers in each sheet have a complex spiral pattern that winds around the atria and ventricles. Cardiac muscle cells form a three-dimensional anastomosing network whereby intercalated discs link almost all cells.

9.5.3 Epicardium

The epicardium covers the heart and comprises a single layer of squamous epithelial cells, their basement membrane and loose connective tissue which attaches it to the underlying myocardium. Coronary blood vessels supply blood to the heart and lie in the epicardium, in which fat cells may be present in large numbers. The epicardium is the inner visceral layer of the pericardium and is continuous with the outer parietal layer and they enclose a potential space, the pericardial cavity. The secretion of minute amounts of fluid into the pericardial cavity by the squamous epithelial cells reduces the friction between visceral and parietal layer of the pericardial cavity when the heart beats.

9.5.4 Electrical conduction system

The electrical conduction system of the heart transmits signals generated by the sinoatrial node to cause contraction of the heart muscle. The pacemaking signal generated in the sinoatrial node travels through the right atrium to the atrioventricular node, along the Bundle of His and through bundle branches (containing the Purkinje fibers) to cause contraction of the heart muscle. This signal stimulates contraction first of the right and left atrium, and then the right and left ventricles. This process allows blood to be pumped throughout the body. (Fig. 9-8)

The Purkinje fibers are located in the inner ventricular walls of the heart, in the subendocardial layer of the endocardium. The Purkinje fibers are specialised conducting fibers larger than cardiomyocytes with fewer myofibrils and a large number of mitochondria that are able to conduct cardiac action potentials more quickly and efficiently than any other cells in the heart. Purkinje fibers allow the heart's conduction system to create synchronized contractions of its ventricles, and are therefore essential for maintaining a consistent heart rhythm.

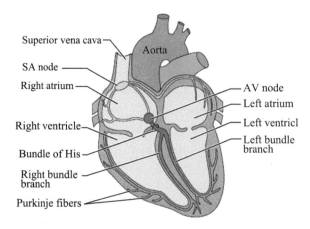

Superior vena cava
Aorta
SA node
Right atrium
AV node
Left atrium
Right ventricle
Left ventricl
Bundle of His
Left bundle branch
Right bundle branch
Purkinje fibers

Fig. 9-8 **Diagram of the electrical conduction system of the heart**

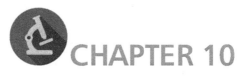

CHAPTER 10
IMMUNE SYSTEM

The immune system is responsible for the immunological defense of the body. The system comprises immune cells, lymphoid tissues and lymphoid organs. The functions of the immune system include:

♦ Immunologic defense: The cells in immune system can recognize and remove antigens as foreign macromolecules or microorganisms that invade into the body.

♦ Immunologic surveillance: The cells in immune system can remove body cells with changed surface antigens such as malignant cells and virus-infected cells.

♦ Immunologic homeostasis: The cells in immune system can remove aging, dead and damaged cells.

Immune system consists mainly of immune cells, lymphoid tissue and lymphoid organs.

10.1 Immune Cells

Immune cells comprise lymphocytes (see chapter 5), antigen presenting cells, dendritic cells, macrophages and mononuclear phagocyte system, etc.

10.1.1 Antigen presenting cells (APCs)

APCs phagocytose, catabolize, and process antigens, form a peptide-MHC II (major histocompatibility II, a type macromolecule) complex and then present the complex to T cells for their activation. APCs are vital for effective adaptive immune response, as the functioning of both cytotoxic and helper T cells is dependent on APCs. (Fig. 10-1)

APCs comprise macrophages, dendritic cells, and non-monocyte-derived APCs (e. g. B cells). Dendritic cells have dendritic processes and MHC-II molecules and can serve as APCs. Dendritic cells are widely distributed through the body: in blood & lymph, epidermis, epithelium of the digestive tract, lymphoid tissue and organs, interstitial stroma of heart, liver, lungs and kidneys.

10.1.2 Macrophages and mononuclear phagocyte system(MPS)

This is the collection of phagocytes, derived from monocytes. All members of the mononuclear phagocyte system arise from a common stem cell in the bone marrow, possess lysosomes, are capable of phagocytosis. Monocytes develop in the bone marrow and circulate in the blood. At the proper signal, they leave the bloodstream by migrating through the endothelium of capillaries or venules. They are widely distributed through the body, including: monocytes in the blood and bone marrow; macrophages in connective tissue, lymphoid tissue, peritoneal and pleural cavities and lungs (dust cells); Kupffer cells in the liver; osteoclasts in the bone; microglial cells of the nerve tissue and Langerhans cells in the skin.

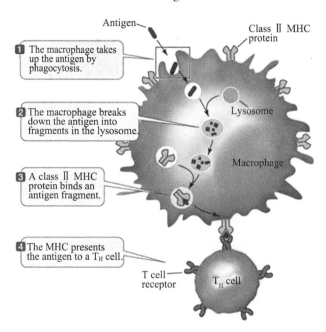

Antigen

Class II MHC protein

1 The macrophage takes up the antigen by phagocytosis.

2 The macrophage breaks down the antigen into fragments in the lysosome.

Lysosome

3 A class II MHC protein binds an antigen fragment.

Macrophage

4 The MHC presents the antigen to a T_H cell.

T cell receptor

T_H cell

Fig. 10-1　Diagram of antigen presenting cell

10.2　Lymphoid Tissue

The main constituents of lymphoid tissue are aggregates of lymphocytes and other cells of the mononuclear phagocyte system. These cells are enmeshed in a supportive framework (stroma) of reticular cells and fibers, so lymphoid tissue is classified as a specialized reticular connective tissue. They are distributed in immune organs including bone marrow, lymph nodes, thymus, and spleen.

There are two formats of lymphoid tissue: diffuse lymphoid tissue and lymphoid nodules. (Fig. 10-2)

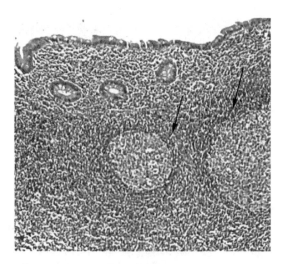

Fig. 10-2　Section of lymphoid tissue: diffuse lymphoid tissue and lymphoid nodules (arrows)

I. Diffuse lymphoid tissue

Diffuse lymphoid tissue is a collection of lymphocytes enmeshed in the reticular cells and fibers, with no clear boundary. T and B lymphocytes are present in this area.

II. Lymphoid nodule

A lymphoid nodule is the spherical or ovoid collections of densely packed lymphocytes (mainly B cells, also Th cells, macrophages).

i. Primary lymphoid nodule

Primary nodules are spherical aggregates of tightly packed B cells in a meshwork of reticular fibers. They are small and isoformed, with no germinal center.

ii. Secondary nodule

After antigen stimulation, the lymphocytes undergo the proliferation by mitosis; primary nodule becomes larger with germinal center, called the secondary nodule. The germinal center is divided into dark zone and light zone, and the latter is covered by a cap. B cells proliferate and differentiate in this center. Germinal centers contain follicular dendritic cells, which trap antigens-antibody complexes and retain these antigens for a long period on their membrane to activate B cells.

10.3   Lymphoid Organs

There are two categories of lymphoid organs: primary and secondary. Primary lymphoid organs (bone marrow and thymus) participate in the development of immunocompetent lymphocytes. Secondary lymphoid organs (lymph nodes, spleen, tonsils, and diffuse lymphoid tissue) function in removing the antigens.

10.3.1   Thymus

Thymus is a primary lymphoid organ that is the site of maturation of T lymphocytes. It is situated in the superior mediastinum, encapsulated by connective tissue and composed of two lobes. The T lymphocytes that enter the thymus become instructed to achieve immunological competence.

The capsule of the thymus is dense irregular collagenous connective tissue, sending septa into the lobes, subdividing them into incomplete lobules. Each lobule is composed of a cortex and a medulla, although the medullae of adjacent lobules are confluent with each other. (Fig. 10-3)

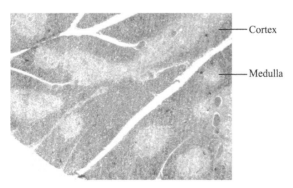

Cortex

Medulla

Fig. 10-3   Section of thymus (low magnification)

Ⅰ. Cortex

The cortex of the thymus appears much darker than does the medulla because of the presence of a large number of T lymphocytes (thymocytes). Immunologically incompetent T cells leave the bone marrow and migrate to the periphery of the thymic cortex, where they undergo extensive proliferation and instruction to become immunocompetent T cells. In addition to the thymocytes, the cortex houses macrophages, dendritic cells, and epithelial reticular cells (thymic epithelial cells).

The capillaries of the cortex are of the continuous type, possess a thick basal lamina, and are invested by a sheath of epithelial reticular cells that form a blood-thymus barrier. Thus, the developing T cells of the cortex are protected from contacting blood-borne macromolecules. However, self-macromolecules are permitted to cross the blood-thymus barrier (probably controlled by the epithelial reticular cells), possibly to eliminate those T cells that are programmed against self-antigens. (Fig. 10-4)

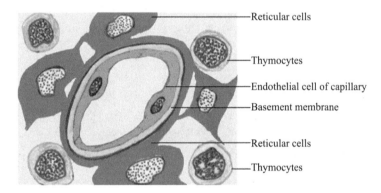

Fig. 10-4　Diagram of blood-thymus barrier

Ⅱ. Medulla

The thymic medulla stains much lighter than the cortex because it has less lymphocytes and has a certain amount of macrophages, dendritic cells, a small population of B cells, and a large number of endothelial-cell-derived epithelial reticular cells.

The medulla is characterized by the presence of Hassall corpuscles. These large, pale-staining cells are arranged around each other, forming whorl-shaped thymic corpuscles (Hassall corpuscles), whose numbers increase with age (Fig. 10-5). The function of thymic corpuscles is not understood completely, although they might be the site of T lymphocyte cell death in the medulla. Epithelial reticular cells of Hassall corpuscles manufacture thymic stromal lymphopoietin.

The primary function of the thymus is to instruct immunoincompetent T cells to achieve immunocompetence. All thymocytes of the medulla are immunocompetent T cells.

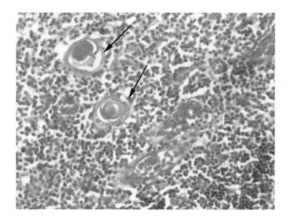

Fig. 10-5   Medulla of thymus(arrows: Hassall corpuscles)

10.3.2   Lymph nodes

Lymph nodes are bean-shaped lymphoid organs, 2 ~ 20 mm in diameter; 500 ~ 600 nodes are found in the body. They are seen along lymphatic vessels. They occur, often as chains or groups, in strategic regions such as the neck, groin, mesenteries, axillae, and abdomen.

An outer capsule of dense fibrous connective tissue that typically merges with surrounding tissues and fat invests each node. It sends delicate, radiating partitions called trabeculae into the interior of the nodes via hilum (Fig. 10-6). The parenchyma of a lymph node contains an outer cortex and an inner medulla.

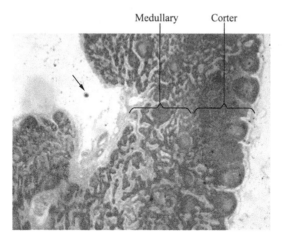

Fig. 10-6   Section of the lymph node(arrow: hilum)

I . Cortex

The darkly stained cortex just under the capsule consists of lymphoid nodules, paracortex and cortical sinuses. (Fig. 10-7)

i . Lymphoid nodules

Both primary and secondary lymphoid nodules are present in the cortex. B cells occupy lymphoid nodules in the cortex.

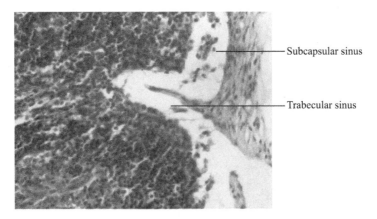

Subcapsular sinus

Trabecular sinus

Fig. 10-7　Cortical lymphatic sinuses of the lymph node

ii . Paracortex

The diffused lymphoid tissue between adjacent lymphoid nodules and between cortex and the medulla is the paracortex. It houses mostly T cells and fibroblastic reticular cells and is the thymus-dependent zone of the lymph node.

Postcapillary venules, with high epithelial cells lining the lumen, are located in the paracortex. Lymphocytes leave the vascular supply by migrating between the cuboidal cells of this unusual endothelium and enter the lymph node.

iii. Cortical sinuses

Cortical sinuses comprise subcapsular sinuses and paratrabecular sinuses. The afferent lymph vessels pierce the capsule on the convex surface of the node and empty their lymph into the subcapsular sinus, which is located just deep to the capsule. This sinus is continuous with the paratrabecular sinuses that parallel the trabeculae and deliver the lymph into the medullary sinuses, eventually to enter the efferent lymphatic vessels. The sinuses are lined with simple squamous epithelium. Within the sinuses, is formed a network of stellate reticular cells whose processes contact those of other cells and the endothelial cells. Macrophages are present to actively phagocytose foreign particulate matter.

II . Medulla

The medulla is composed of lymphoid cells that are organized in clusters known as medullary cords, surrounded by large, tortuous lymph sinuses (medullary sinus). (Fig. 10-8)

i . Medullary cords

The cells of the medullary cords (lymphocytes, plasma cells, and macrophages) are enmeshed in a network of reticular fibers and reticular cells. The lymphocytes migrate from the cortex to enter the medullary sinuses from which they enter the efferent lymphatic vessels to leave the lymph node. Histological sections of the medulla also display the presence of trabeculae, arising from the thickened capsule of the hilum, conveying blood vessels into and out of the lymph node.

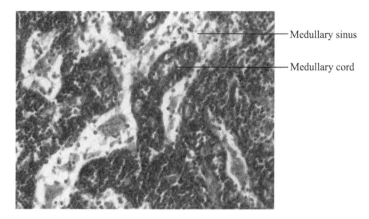

Fig. 10-8   Medulla of the lymph node

ii . Medullary sinuses

Structurally, medullary sinuses are the same as cortical sinuses. They receive the lymph from the cortex and drain into the efferent lymphatic vessels in hilum.

Ⅲ. Functions

The functions of lymph nodes include:

i . Filter lymph fluid

Lymph percolates slowly through the tortuous sinuses, maximizing the time available for macrophages to remove antigens, foreign particles, and other debris. The route of lymph fluid is shown in Fig. 10-9.

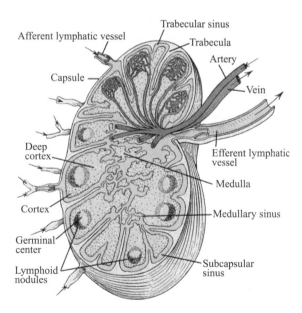

Fig. 10-9   The route of lymph fluid in a lymph node

ii . Sites for immune responses

Under stimulation of antigens, both B and T cells proliferate and produce antibodies and effector T cells causing humoral and cellular immunity, respectively.

iii. Recirculation of lymphocytes

Lymphocytes circulate repeatedly from lymphoid tissue and organs through the lymphatic vessels and into the bloodstream. The most actively recirculating cells are memory cells of both T and B cells. The route is: lymphocytes in the blood stream cross the wall of postcapillary venules into the lymphoid tissue. Lymphocytes in the lymphoid tissue enter lymphatic vessels, then into the bloodstream. This recirculation increase the probability of meeting antigens, distribute information concerning antigens, and unite the different parts of the immune system.

10.3.3 Spleen

Spleen is the largest lymphoid organ in the body, located in the peritoneum in the upper left quadrant of the abdominal cavity. Its dense irregular connective tissue capsule, occasionally housing smooth muscle cells, give rise to trabeculae extending to interior of the spleen. The simple squamous epithelium of the peritoneum covers the spleen.

The parenchyma spleen consists of white pulp and red pulp. (Fig. 10-10, Fig. 10-11)

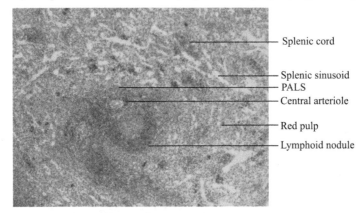

Splenic cord

Splenic sinusoid
PALS
Central arteriole

Red pulp

Lymphoid nodule

Fig. 10-10　Section of the spleen

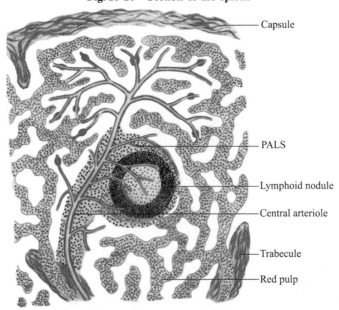

Capsule

PALS

Lymphoid nodule

Central arteriole

Trabecule

Red pulp

Fig. 10-11　Diagram of the spleen

I . White pulp

White pulp is the grayish white islands of lymphoid tissue in fresh, comprising periarteriolar lymphatic sheaths (PALS) and lymphoid nodules.

i . Periarteriolar lymphatic sheaths (PALS)

The central arteriole is derived from the splenic artery after many treelike branchings. Surrounding a central arteriole, the diffuse lymphoid tissue forms periarteriolar lymphatic sheaths (PALS). T cells are found mainly in PALS around the central arteriole.

ii . Lymphoid nodules

In white pulp, lymphoid nodules lie in more peripheral relative to the arterioles. As in lymph nodes, B cells may be found in primary lymphoid nodules or secondary nodules with germinal centers.

Surrounding white pulp is a shell of sparsely cellular lymphoid tissue, the marginal zone, which contains many macrophages and some B lymphocytes. This zone is not as well defined in humans.

II . Red pulp

Red pulp makes up most of the spleen parenchyma, its color being due mostly to abundant erythrocytes. It consists of splenic sinusoids and splenic cords (Billroth cords). Red pulp resembles a sponge in that the spaces within the sponge represent the sinuses and the material among the spaces denotes the splenic cords. (Fig. 10-12)

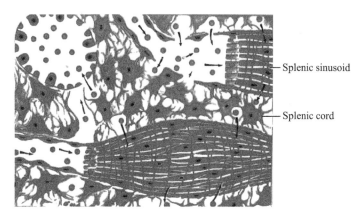

Fig. 10-12   Red pulp

i . Splenic sinuses

The endothelial lining cells of splenic sinuses are fusiform, with large gap between two adjacent cells. The sinuses are surrounded by reticular fibers that wrap around the sinuses as individual thin strands of thread. The reticular fibers are arranged perpendicular to the longitudinal axis of the sinuses. Flexible blood cells pass from splenic cords to the lumen of the sinusoids.

ii . Splenic cords

The splenic cords are composed of a loose network of reticular fibers, and many closely packed fixed or wandering cells, including reticular cells, lymphocytes, plasma cells, macrophages, and all formed elements of circulating blood are seen in the cords.

iii. Blood supply

The splenic artery branches repeatedly as it pierces the connective tissue capsule at the hilum of the spleen. Branches of these vessels form trabecular arteries, which go in the trabeculae decreasing sizes, and finally leave the trabeculae. These vessels are central arterioles, surrounded by PALS. Branches of the central arteriole, are known as follicular arterioles. At its termination, the central artery loses its lymphatic sheath and subdivides into several short parallel branches, known as penicillar arteries, which enter the red pulp. Splenic sinuses are drained by small veins of the pulp, which are tributaries of larger and larger veins that merge to form the splenic vein, a tributary of the portal vein.

iv. Functions

The spleen functions not only in T-cell and B-cell proliferation and immune response but also as a filter of the blood and in destroying old erythrocytes and old platelets. During fetal development, the spleen is a hemopoietic organ; if necessary, it can resume that function in an adult. Moreover, splenic sinuses can store some amount of blood.

10.3.4 Mucosa-associated lymphoid tissue (MALT)

Mucous membranes (or mucosa) of the gastrointestinal, respiratory, and genitourinary tracts are open to the external environment, so they harbor the body's largest, most diverse populations of microorganisms and pathogens. Extensive mucosal surfaces lead to vulnerability to infection. The diffuse lymphoid tissue in the lamina propria of these membranes is known as MALT. MALT may be subdivided into gut-associated lymphoid tissue (GALT), bronchus-associated lymphoid tissue (BALT), nose-associated lymphoid tissue (NALT), and vulvovaginal-associated (VALT) lymphoid tissue. GALT includes tonsils, Peyer's patches, appendix, and less organized lymphocyte infiltrations scattered along the gastrointestinal tract.

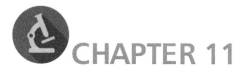

CHAPTER 11
RESPIRATORY SYSTEM

The respiratory system is composed of a sequence of airways and the lungs. The function of the respiratory system is to transport gases between the atmosphere and the lungs where gas exchange between air and blood occurs. Oxygen diffuses into blood in capillaries in the lungs and carbon dioxide is released from the blood.

The respiratory system is subdivided into two major components: the conducting portion and the respiratory portion. The conducting portion situated both outside and within the lungs, conveys air from the external milieu to the lungs. The respiratory portion, within the lungs, functions in the actual exchange of oxygen and carbon dioxide.

The respiratory tract, the passage of the air, is divided into an upper and a lower respiratory tract. The upper tract includes the nasal cavities, pharynx and the part of the larynx above the vocal folds. The lower tract includes the lower part of the larynx, the trachea and bronchi. When bronchi enter into the lungs, they go on branching and form the intrapulmonary tracheobronchial tree.

11.1　Trachea

The trachea is a tube that begins at the cricoid cartilage of the larynx and ends when it bifurcates to form the primary bronchi. The wall of the trachea is reinforced by C-shaped cartilage rings. The open ends of these rings face posteriorly and are connected to each other by smooth muscle. Because of this arrangement of the C-rings, the trachea is rounded anteriorly but flattened posteriorly. The trachea has three layers: mucosa, submucosa, and adventitia. (Fig. 11-1)

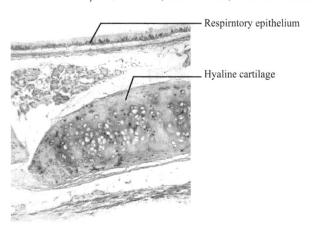

Respirntory epithelium

Hyaline cartilage

Fig. 11-1　Section of the trachea

11.1.1 Mucosa

The mucosal lining of the trachea is composed of pseudostratified ciliated columnar (respiratory) epithelium, the subepithelial connective tissue (lamina propria), and a relatively thick bundle of elastic fibers separating the mucosa from the submucosa.

I. Respiratory epithelium

The respiratory epithelium, a pseudostratified ciliated columnar epithelium, rests on a thick basement membrane. The epithelium is composed of five cell types: ciliated columnar cells, goblet cells, basal cells, brush cells, and cells of the diffuse neuroendocrine system (DNES). All of these cells come into contact with the basement membrane. (Fig. 11-2)

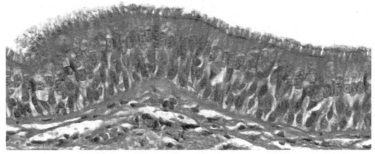

(a) Section of trachea showing respiratory epithelium

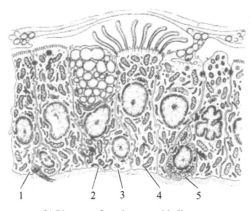

(b) Piagram of respiratory epithelium

1—Brush cell; 2—Goblet cell; 3—basal cell; 4—Ciliated columnar cell; 5—DENS cell

Fig. 11-2　Diagram of the respiratory epithelium

i. Ciliated columnar cells

They constitute about 30% of the total respiratory epithelial cell population. These tall, slender cells have a basally located nucleus and possess cilia on their apical cell membrane. The cilia move the mucus and its trapped particulate matter, via ciliary wavy action, toward the nasopharynx for elimination.

ii. Goblet cells

They constitute about 30% of the total cell population of the respiratory epithelium. They produce mucinogen, which becomes hydrated and is known as mucin when released into an aqueous environment and this traps particulate matter which may be harmful. Once the mucin is mixed with other material in the watery environment, it is known as mucus.

iii. Basal cells

The short basal cells are located on the basement membrane, but their apical surfaces do not reach the lumen. These relatively undifferentiated cells are considered to be stem cells that proliferate to replace goblet, ciliated columnar, and brush cells.

iv. Brush cells

Brush cells are narrow, columnar cells with microvilli. Their function is unknown, but they have been associated with nerve endings, suggesting that they may have a sensory role.

v. DNES cells

These cells are also known as small-granule cells. Many of these cells possess long, slender processes that extend into the lumen, and it is suggested that they have the ability to monitor the oxygen and carbon dioxide levels in the lumen of the airway. These cells are closely associated with naked sensory nerve endings. DNES cells contain numerous granules, which house pharmacological agents such as amines, polypeptides, acetylcholine, serotonin, and adenosine triphosphate. Under hypoxic conditions, these agents are released not only into the synaptic clefts but also into the connective tissue spaces of the lamina propria, where they act as paracrine hormones or may enter the vascular supply to act as hormones.

II. Lamina propria

The lamina propria of the trachea is composed of a loose, fibroelastic connective tissue. It contains lymphoid elements (e. g. lymphoid nodules, lymphocytes, and neutrophils) as well as mucous and seromucous glands, whose ducts open onto the epithelial surface. A dense layer of elastic fibers, the elastic lamina, separates the lamina propria from the underlying submucosa.

11.1.2   Submucosa

The tracheal submucosa is composed of a dense, irregular fibroelastic connective tissue housing numerous mucous and seromucous glands. The short ducts of these glands pierce the elastic lamina and the lamina propria to open onto the epithelial surface. Lymphoid elements are also present in the submucosa. Moreover, this region has a rich blood and lymph supply, the smaller branches of which reach the lamina propria.

11.1.3   Adventitia

The adventitia of the trachea is composed of a fibroelastic connective tissue and houses C-shaped rings of hyaline cartilage. The ends of the hyaline cartilage rings are joined with fibrous connective tissue. The adventitia also is responsible for anchoring the trachea to the adjacent structures (i. e. esophagus and connective tissues of the neck).

11.2   Bronchi and Bronchial Tree

The trachea bifurcates into primary bronchi. The structure of the primary bronchi is identical to that of the trachea, except that bronchi are smaller in diameter, and their walls are thinner.

The bronchial tree begins at the bifurcation of the trachea, as the right and left primary bronchi, which form branches that gradually decrease in size. The bronchial tree is composed of airways located outside of the lungs (the primary bronchi, extrapulmonary bronchi) and airways located inside of the lungs: the intrapulmonary bronchi (lobar [secondary]), and their tributary branches.

Each primary bronchus, accompanied by the pulmonary arteries, veins, and lymph vessels, pierces the root (hilum) of the lung and will be further branched in the lungs. (Fig. 11-3)

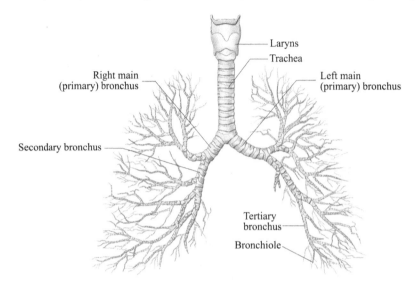

Fig. 11-3   Diagram of the bronchial tree

11.3   Lungs

Two lungs are situated within the thoracic cavity of the chest. The primary bronchi, after entering the lungs, branch repeatedly to form the intrapulmonary portion of the bronchial tree, at end portion of which alveoli are connected. The intrapulmonary portion of the bronchial tree constitutes the parenchyma of the lungs, which is divided into the conducting and respiratory portion.

11.3.1   Conducting portion

This portion comprises intrapulmonary bronchi (lobar [secondary bronchi]), segmental [tertiary] bronchi, bronchioles, and terminal bronchioles. The bronchial tree divides 15 to 20 times before reaching the level of terminal bronchioles. As the airways progressively decrease in size, several trends are observed, including a decrease in all of the following: the amount of cartilage, the numbers of glands and goblet cells, and the height of epithelial cells. Also, there is an increase in smooth muscle and elastic tissue with respect to the thickness of the wall.

I . Secondary (lobar) bronchus

The right bronchus trifurcates to lead to the three lobes of the right lung, and the left bronchus bifurcates, sending branches to the two lobes of the left lung. Each secondary (lobar) bronchus is the airway to a lobe of the lung. The left lung has two lobes and thus has two secondary bronchi; the right lung has three lobes and thus has three secondary bronchi. Their histological characteristics are similar to primary bronchi, except that the cartilage rings are replaced by irregular plates of hyaline cartilage and become sparser.

II . Tertiary (segmental) bronchi

As secondary bronchi enter the lobes of the lung, they subdivide into smaller branches, tertiary (segmental) bronchi (Fig. 11-4). Each tertiary bronchus arborizes and leads to a discrete section of lung tissue, known as a bronchopulmonary segment. Each lung has 10 bronchopulmonary segments that are completely separated from one another by connective tissue elements and are clinically important in surgical procedures involving the lungs. As the arborized branches of intrapulmonary bronchi decrease in diameter, they eventually lead to bronchioles.

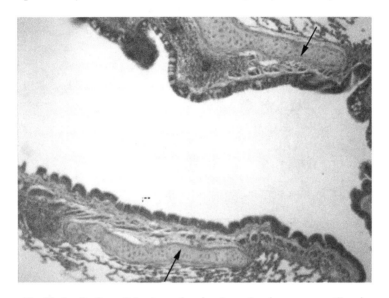

Fig. 11-4   Section of the lung showing bronchus(arrows: cartilage)

III. Bronchioles

Bronchioles possess no cartilage in their walls, are smaller than 1 mm in diameter, and have Clara cells in their epithelial lining. Each bronchiole supplies air to a pulmonary lobule. The epithelial lining of bronchioles ranges from ciliated simple columnar with occasional goblet cells in larger bronchioles to simple cuboidal with occasional Clara cells, and no goblet cells in smaller bronchioles.

Clara cells are columnar with domeshaped apices that have short blunt microvilli. Their apical cytoplasm houses numerous secretory granules containing glycoproteins. These cells protect the bronchiolar epithelium by lining it with their secretory product.

IV. Terminal bronchioles

Terminal bronchioles form the smallest and most distal region of the conducting portion of the respiratory system. Each bronchiole subdivides to form several smaller terminal bronchioles, which are smaller than 0. 5 mm in diameter. The epithelium of terminal bronchioles is composed of Clara cells and cuboidal cells. The lamina propria consists of fibroelastic connective tissue and is surrounded by one or two layers of smooth muscle cells. Terminal bronchioles branch to give rise to respiratory bronchioles. (Fig. 11-5)

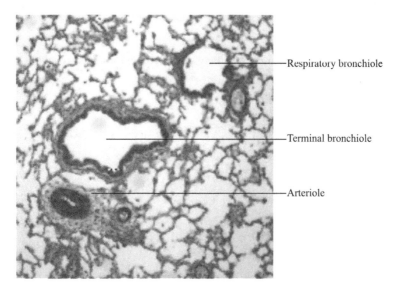

Respiratory bronchiole

Terminal bronchiole

Arteriole

Fig. 11-5   Section of the lung showing terminal bronchioles, respiratory bronchiole and arteriole

11.3.2   Respiratory portion

This portion includes respiratory bronchioles, alveolar ducts, alveolar sacs, and alveoli. This is the site exchange of gases occurs. (Fig. 11-5, Fig. 11-6)

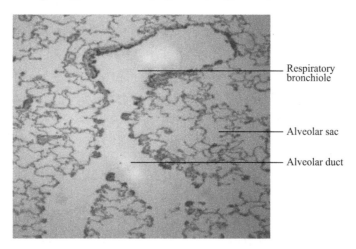

Respiratory bronchiole

Alveolar sac

Alveolar duct

Fig. 11-6   Section of the lung showing respiratory portion of the bronchial tree

I. Respiratory bronchioles

Respiratory bronchioles are the first region of the respiratory system where exchange of gases can occur. The walls of respiratory bronchioles are not complete. Rather they are broken up by the thin-walled, pouch-like structures, alveoli, composed of an attenuated simple squamous epithelium. As respiratory bronchioles branch, they become narrower in diameter, and their population of alveoli increases. Subsequent to several branchings, each respiratory bronchiole terminates in an alveolar duct.

II. Alveolar ducts and alveolar sacs

Alveolar ducts do not have walls of their own; they are merely a continuous sequence of alveoli. An alveolar duct that arises from a respiratory bronchiole forms branches, and each of the resultant alveolar ducts usually ends as a blind outpouching composed of two or more small clusters of alveoli, in which each cluster is known as an alveolar sac. These alveolar sacs thus open into a common space.

III. Alveoli

Alveoli are small, cup-shaped outpocketings of respiratory bronchioles, alveolar ducts, and sacs that are like closely-packed cells of a honeycomb. Very slender partitions, the interalveolar septa, separate adjacent alveoli. (Fig. 11-7)

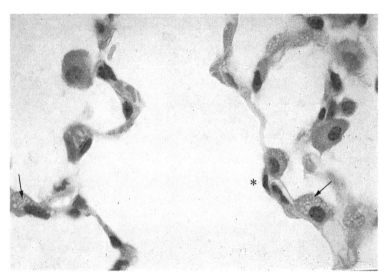

Fig. 11-7   Section of the lung showing alveoli
(asterisk: type I pneumocyte; arrows: type II pneumocytes)

i. Pneumocytes

Alveoli have a continuous lining of simple squamous epithelium. Two types of cells in this epithelium are the type I and the type II pneumocytes. (Fig. 11-7)

♦ Type I pneumocytes: Type I cells are flattened and possess a large surface area to facilitate gas exchange. They have elongated, darkly stained nucleuses. Type I pneumocytes cover about 95% of the alveolar surface, even though they constitute only 40% of all the epithelial cells.

♦ Type II pneumocytes: Type II pneumocytes take up 60% of cells lining the alveoli, however, just accounting for only 5% of the lining cells. They are roughly spherical cells, with a centrally placed nucleus, rich in RER, a well-developed Golgi apparatus, and mitochondria. The most distinguishing feature of these cells is the presence of membrane-bound lamellar bodies that contain pulmonary surfactant. The surfactant reduces surface tension in the alveoli. During inspiration, this low surface tension makes it easier to draw air into the alveoli and helps to prevent the alveoli from collapsing.

ii. Interalveolar septa

Interalveolar septa is the sparse connective tissue around alveoli and consists of capillaries, elastin fibres, alveolar macrophages and a little collagen.

◆ Capillaries: Interalveolar septa is rich in continuous capillaries. In some regions there is no connective tissue and the basement membranes of an alveolar epithelium and the adjacent capillary endothelium are fused, thus reducing the distance gases have to travel between air and blood.

◆ Elastin fibres: The elastin fibres are stretched on inspiration and this helps to draw air into the alveoli. Importantly, recoil of the elastin during expiration helps to expel air from the alveoli.

◆ Kohn pore: Pores present in the interalveolar septa are known as Kohn pores. The air spaces of the two alveoli may communicate with each other through the Kohn pores. These pores function to equilibrate air pressure within pulmonary segments.

◆ Alveolar macrophages (dust cells): They are derived from the monocytes of the blood, phagocytose inhaled particulate matter and microorganisms, and thus maintain a sterile environment within the lungs.

Gas exchange between blood and air occurs across the **blood-air barrier**, which is readily permeable to gases via diffusion. It comprises the thin layer of surfactant produced by type II pneumocytes, type I pneumocytes lining the alveolus, the endothelium of the continuous capillaries, and their fused basal laminae. (Fig. 11-8)

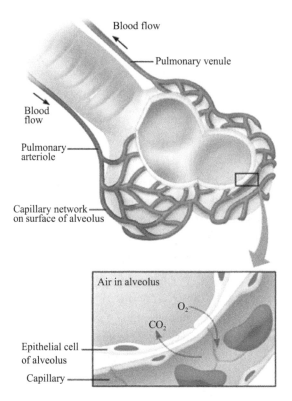

Fig. 11-8   Diagram of blood-air barrier

11.3.3 Pulmonary vascular supply

The pulmonary arteries supply deoxygenated blood to the lungs. Branches of these vessels follow the bronchial tubes into the lobules of the lung. When they reach the respiratory bronchioles, these vessels form an extensive pulmonary capillary network. The blood in the capillary bed becomes oxygenated and then drains into veins of increasing diameter. These tributaries of the pulmonary vein carry oxygenated blood and travel in the septa between lobules of the lung. Thus, the veins follow a path that is different from that of the arteries, until they reach the apex of the lobule, where they accompany the bronchial tubes to the hilus of the lung to deliver oxygenated blood to the heart.

Bronchial arteries, which are branches of the thoracic aorta, bring nutrient-laden and oxygen-laden blood to the bronchial tree, interlobular septa, and pleura of the lungs. Many of the small branches anastomose with those of the pulmonary system. Others are drained by tributaries of the bronchial veins.

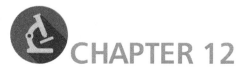

CHAPTER 12
DIGESTIVE TRACT

The digestive tract, or the alimentary canal, is the tract from the mouth to anus. It is the place that food is churned, liquefied, and digested; its nutritional elements and water are absorbed; and its indigestible components are eliminated. The digestive tract is divided into the mouth, esophagus, stomach, small intestine (duodenum, jejunum, and ileum), and large intestine (cecum, colon, rectum, anal canal, and appendix).

The structure of the digestive tract is related to its functions and different aspects of function occur at different locations along the tract, yet they have some common structural characteristics.

12.1　General Structures of the Digestive Tract

Generally, the digestive tract is composed of the following layers: mucosa, submucosa, muscularis externa, and serosa (adventitia). (Fig. 12-1)

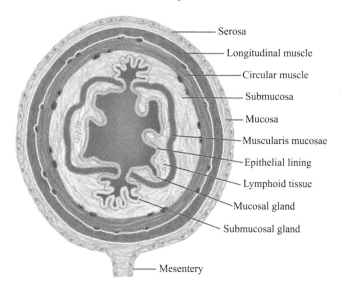

Fig. 12-1　**General structures of the digestive tract**

I . Mucosa

The lumen of the digestive tract is lined by a mucosa, which consists of an epithelium, connective tissue lamina propria and a layer of smooth muscle forming the muscularis mucosae. The epithelium of the mucosa reflects the primary function(s) occurring in that region, deep to which is a loose connective tissue known as the lamina propria. This connective tissue houses glands as well as blood and lymph vessels and occasional lymphoid nodules. The mucosa is important in forming a barrier between substances ingested, including microorganisms, and the internal environment of the body. In regions where the muscularis mucosae is present, contraction of this muscle moves and folds the mucosa, aiding contact between the contents of the lumen and the surface epithelial cells.

II. Submucosa

The mucosa is surrounded by a dense, irregular fibroelastic connective tissue layer, the submucosa. This layer houses glands in the esophagus and duodenum. The submucosa also contains blood and lymph vessels as well as a component of the enteric nervous system known as Meissner plexus. This plexus, which also houses postganglionic parasympathetic nerve cell bodies, controls the motility of the mucosa, submucosa, and the secretory activities of its glands.

III. Muscularis externa

The muscularis externa is usually composed of inner circular and outer longitudinal smooth muscle layers, responsible for peristaltic activity, which moves the contents of the lumen along the alimentary tract. A second component of the enteric nervous system, known as the Auerbach plexus, is situated between these two muscle layers and regulates the activity of the muscularis externa (and, to a limited extent, the activity of the mucosa). The Auerbach plexus also houses postganglionic parasympathetic nerve cell bodies.

IV. Adventitia

The muscularis externa is enveloped by a thin connective tissue layer known as adventitia. The adventitia may or may not be surrounded by the simple squamous epithelium of the visceral peritoneum. If the region of the digestive tract is intraperitoneal, it is invested by peritoneum, and the covering is known as the serosa. If the organ is retroperitoneal, it adheres to the body wall by its dense irregular connective tissue component and is known as the fibrosa.

12.2 Mouth

The mouth (oral cavity) contains the tongue and teeth. The epithelium of the mucosa lining the cheeks and tongue is able to resist the wear and tear involved in chewing food, and in most regions it is a nonkeratinized stratified squamous epithelium. This epithelial surface is moistened by secretions from small serous and mucous glands in the submucosal layer and from salivary glands which drain their saliva into the oral cavity. Physical breakdown of food occurs in the mouth and it is mixed with salivary gland secretions.

12.3 Esophagus

The esophagus is a muscular tube that conveys the bolus (masticated food) from the oral pharynx to the stomach. Its mucosa presents numerous longitudinal folds with intervening grooves that cause the lumen to appear to be obstructed; however, when the esophagus is distended, the folds disappear. (Fig. 12-2, Fig. 12-3)

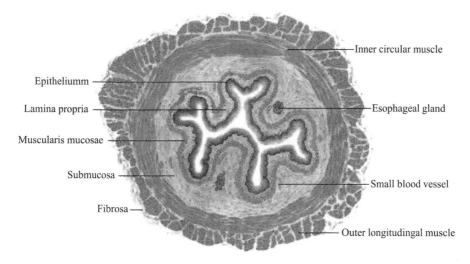

Inner circular muscle

Epitheliumm

Lamina propria

Muscularis mucosae

Submucosa

Fibrosa

Esophageal gland

Small blood vessel

Outer longitudingal muscle

Fig. 12-2   Transverse section of esophagus(low magnification)

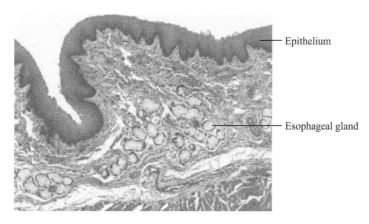

Epithelium

Esophageal gland

Fig. 12-3   Section of esophagus(middle magnification)

Ⅰ. Mucosa

The esophageal mucosa is composed of a stratified squamous epithelium, fibroelastic lamina propria, and a longitudinal smooth muscle which compose the muscularis mucosae.

Ⅱ. Submucosa

The submucosa of the esophagus houses mucous glands known as the esophageal glands proper. The submucosa of the esophagus is composed of a dense fibroelastic connective tissue, which houses the esophageal glands. These tubuloacinar glands are mainly composed of mucous cells.

Ⅲ. Muscularis externa

The muscularis externa of the esophagus is composed of both skeletal and smooth muscle cells. The muscularis externa of the esophagus is arranged in the two orientations, inner circular and outer longitudinal. However, these muscle layers are unusual in that they are composed of both skeletal and smooth muscle fibers. The muscularis externa of the upper third has mostly skeletal muscle, the middle third has both skeletal and smooth muscle, and the lowest third has only smooth muscle fibers.

IV. Adventitia

The esophagus is covered by a fibrosa until it pierces the diaphragm, after which it is covered by a serosa.

12.4 Stomach

The stomach is a dilated portion of the gastrointestinal tract. It has four regions: the cardia, the fundus, the body and the pylorus (Fig. 12-4). The cardiac region is continuous with the lower end of the esophagus. The fundus is the part of the stomach lying closest to the diaphragm. The body of the stomach is the largest part of the stomach and the pylorus connects the body of the stomach to the duodenum. The stomach produces gastric juices, containing mucus, water, hydrochloric acid and enzymes able to digest carbohydrates, fats and proteins. The mixture of gastric juices and ingested food and drink is known as chyme.

Histologically, the fundus and body are identical. All the gastric regions display rugae, longitudinal folds of the mucosa and submucosa. Rugae permit expansion of the stomach as it fills with food and gastric juices.

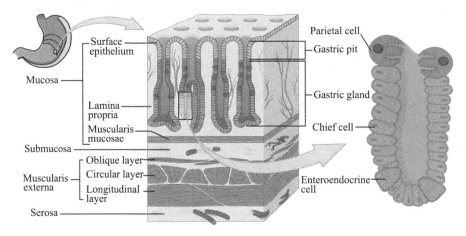

Fig. 12-4 Sections of the stomach

12.4.1 Mucosa

The simple columnar epithelium of the gastric mucosa dips into the lamina propria and forms gastric pits and they secrete mucus. This mucus forms a thick protective layer which helps to ensure that the stomach cells are not damaged by gastric secretions. The base of the pits continues with the gastric glands, which extend as tubes deep into the lamina propria and reach the muscularis mucosae.

I. Gastric glands

Gastric glands have different names depending upon their locations. The gastric glands in the fundus and the body are named as the fundic glands; in the cardiac region are the cardiac glands and in the pyloric region are the pyloric glands.

Each fundic gland extends from the muscularis mucosae to the base of the gastric pit and is subdivided into three regions: isthmus, neck, and base. The fundic gland is composed of five cell types: chief (zymogenic) cells, parietal (oxyntic) cells, mucous neck cells, endocrine cell, and stem cells. (Fig. 12-5, Fig. 12-6)

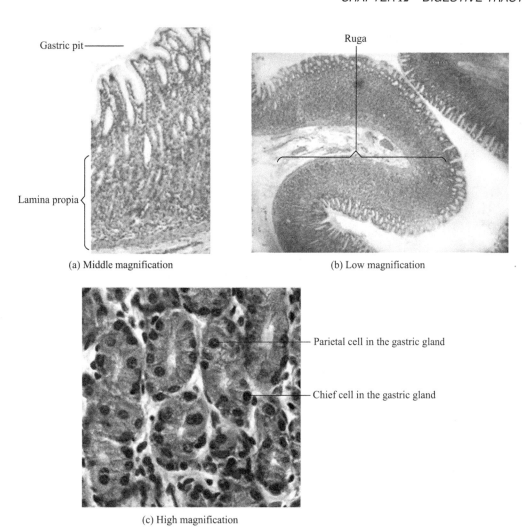

Gastric pit

Lamina propia

(a) Middle magnification

Ruga

(b) Low magnification

Parietal cell in the gastric gland

Chief cell in the gastric gland

(c) High magnification

Fig. 12-5   Section of the stomach

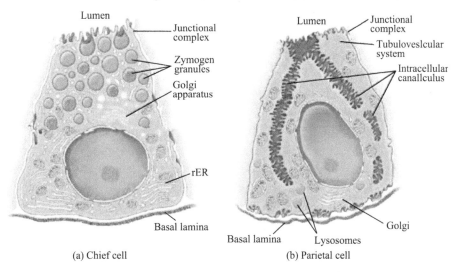

Lumen

Junctional complex

Zymogen granules

Golgi apparatus

rER

Basal lamina

(a) Chief cell

Lumen

Junctional complex

Tubuloveslcular system

Intracellular canallculus

Basal lamina

Lysosomes

Golgi

(b) Parietal cell

Fig. 12-6   Diagram of the two types of the cells in the gastric glands

i . Zymogenic (Chief) cells

They stains basophilic upon HE staining due to the large proportion of rough endoplasmic reticulum in its cytoplasm. They are generally located deep in the mucosal layer of the stomach lining. They produce and secrete pepsinogen and lipase, which digest protein and lipids, respectively. Pepsinogen is inactive until it is converted by the acidity of the gastric juices, into pepsin, which breaks proteins down into smaller molecules. The release of gastric enzymes is stimulated by the vagus nerve, which is part of the parasympathetic nervous system.

ii . Parietal cells

The parietal cells are large, round to pyramid-shaped and located mainly in the upper half of the fundic glands. They have round, basally located nuclei, and their cytoplasm is eosinophilic. The invaginations of their apical plasmalemma form deep intracellular canaliculi lined by microvilli. The cytoplasm bordering these canaliculi is richly filled by round and tubular vesicles, the tubulovesicular system. Additionally, the cell is rich in mitochondria. The number of microvilli and the abundance of the tubulovesicular system are related to each other and vary with the HCl secretory activity of the cell. During active HCl production, the number of microvilli increases, and the tubulovesicular system decreases. Parietal cells manufacture not only HCl but also gastric intrinsic factor. Intrinsic factor is a glycoprotein essential for the absorption of vitamin B_{12}, which is essential for the production of red blood cells. Without intrinsic factor pernicious anaemia develops.

iii . Mucous neck cells

They have basally located nuclei, well-developed Golgi apparatus and rough endoplasmic reticulum (RER). The apical cytoplasm is filled with mucinogen, and when released, will be mixed with and lubricates the chyme, reducing friction as it moves along the digestive tract.

iv . Endocrine cells

These cells secrete a variety of hormones into the local environment and into blood vessels that modify the activity of other cells. For example, some cells secrete gastrin, which stimulates contraction of the muscularis externa of the stomach and relaxation of the pyloric sphincter, thus moving stomach contents into the duodenum.

v . Stem cells

They proliferate to replace all of the specialized cells lining the fundic glands, gastric pits, and luminal surface. Newly formed cells migrate to their new locations either deep into the gland or up into the gastric pit and gastric lining.

II . Differences in the mucosa of the cardiac and pyloric regions

The mucosa of the cardiac region of the stomach differs from that of the fundic region, in that the gastric pits are shallower, and the base of its glands is highly coiled. The cell population of these cardiac glands is composed mostly of surface-lining cells, some mucous neck cells, a few endocrine cells and parietal cells, and no chief cells.

The glands of the pyloric region contain the same cell types as those in the cardiac region, but the predominant cell type in the pylorus is the mucous neck cell. In addition to producing soluble mucus, these cells secrete lysozyme, a bactericidal enzyme. Pyloric glands are highly convoluted and tend to branch. Additionally, the gastric pits of the pyloric region are deeper than in either the cardiac or fundic region.

12.4.2   Submucosa

Submucosa of the stomach is the dense, irregular collagenous connective tissue, rich in vascular and lymphatic network that supplies and drains the vessels of the lamina propria. The cell population of the submucosa resembles that of any connective tissue proper. Meissner plexus can be seen in this layer.

12.4.3   Muscularis externa

The stomach has three layers: an innermost oblique, a middle circular and an outer longitudinal layer. These muscle layers help prevent over distension of the stomach and their contractions help mix the chyme and move it towards the small intestine. In the pyloric region of the stomach, at the gastroduodenal junction, the muscularis externa is thickened and functions as a sphincter. The sphincter is controlled by autonomic nerves and hormones which regulate the passage of chyme into the duodenum.

12.4.4   Adventitia of the stomach

The stomach is covered by a serosal (peritoneal) membrane. The surface squamous epithelial cells of the peritoneal membrane secrete small amounts of fluid (into the peritoneal cavity) and, as the stomach fills with food and drink, it moves relatively easily against adjacent structures. Within the connective tissue of the peritoneal membrane large accumulations of fat cells may be present.

12.5   Small Intestine

The small intestine, the longest region of the digestive tract, has three parts: duodenum, jejunum and ileum. Digestion continues in the small intestine and involves digestive enzymes from secretory cells in the mucosal epithelium. Secretions from the pancreas and liver enter the

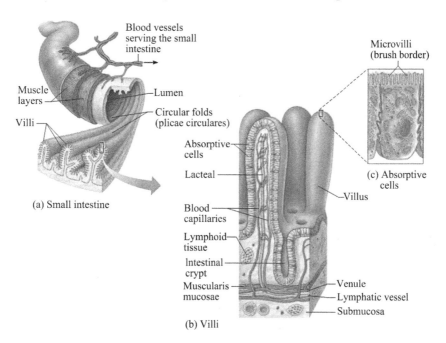

Fig. 12-7   Diagram of small intestine

lumen of the duodenum and these also aid digestion. Most of the products of digestion, e. g. amino acids and monosaccharides, are absorbed across the epithelium lining the small intestine and pass into blood vessels; fatty acids and triglycerides pass into lacteals (small, blind-ended lymph vessels). (Fig. 12-7)

12.5.1 Modifications of the luminal surface

The surface area of the intestinal lumen is enlarged by the formation of plicae circulares, villi, microvilli, and intestinal crypts(Fig. 12-7, Fig. 12-8).

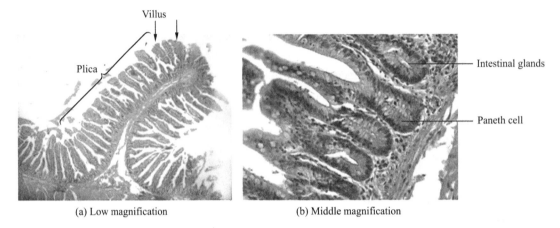

(a) Low magnification   (b) Middle magnification

Fig. 12-8   Section of small intestine

I. Plicae

Plicae circulares (valves of Kerckring) are transverse folds of the submucosa and mucosa that form semicircular to helical elevations. Unlike rugae of the stomach, these are permanent fixtures of the duodenum and jejunum and end in the proximal half of the ileum. They not only increase the surface area but also decrease the velocity of the movement of chyme along the alimentary canal.

II. Villi

Villi are covered by columnar epithelial absorptive cells and goblet cells and have a core of connective tissue supporting blood vessels and lymphatic vessels (lacteals). A few smooth muscle cells are also present in villi and their contractions move the villi amongst the chyme, thus aiding absorption. Villi are more numerous in the duodenum than in the jejunum or the ileum.

III. Microvilli

Microvilli are the modifications of the apical cell membrane of the epithelial cells covering the intestinal villi, increasing the surface area of the small intestine greatly.

Thus, the three types of intestinal surface modifications increase the total surface area available for absorption of nutrients 400 to 600 times. Invaginations of the epithelium into the lamina propria between the villi form intestinal crypts or intestinal glands, which also augment the surface area of the small intestine.

12.5.2 Layers of small intestine

I. Mucosa

The mucosa of the small intestine is composed of the usual three layers: a simple columnar epithelium, the lamina propria, and the muscularis mucosae.

i. Epithelium

The simple columnar epithelium covering the villi and the surface of the intervillar spaces is composed of absorptive cells, goblet cells, and endocrine cells.

A. Surface absorptive cells　Surface absorptive cells, the most numerous cells of the epithelium are tall columnar cells that function in terminal digestion and absorption of water and nutrients. They are tall cells with basally located oval nuclei. Their apical surface presents a striated border, and in good tissue preparations, the presence of terminal bars is also evident. Terminal bar is a histological term given to the group of junctional complexes that attach adjacent epithelial cells on their lateral surfaces. They build up the paracellular barrier of epithelia and seal the paracellular space.

The principal functions of the absorptive cells are terminal digestion and absorption of nutrients and water. Additionally, these cells re-esterify fatty acids into triglycerides, form chylomicrons, and transport them as well as the bulk of the absorbed nutrients into the lamina propria for distribution to the rest of the body.

B. Goblet cells　Goblet cells are unicellular glands. The duodenum has the smallest number of goblet cells, and their number increases toward the ileum. These cells manufacture mucinogen, whose hydrated form is mucin, a component of mucus, a protective layer lining the lumen.

C. Endocrine cells　The small intestine has various types of endocrine cells. The cells produce numerous hormones that affect movement of the small intestine and help regulate gastric HCl secretion and the release of pancreatic secretions.

D. Microfold cells (M cells)　Microfold cells phagocytose and transport antigens from the lumen to the lamina propria. The simple columnar epithelial lining of the small intestine is replaced by squamous-like M cells in regions where lymphoid nodules abut the epithelium. These M cells, which are believed to belong to the mononuclear phagocyte system of cells, which phagocytose, and transport antigens present in the intestinal lumen. (Fig. 12-9)

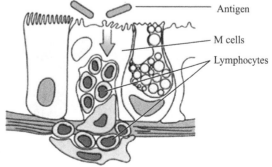

Fig. 12-9　Diagram of a M cell

ii. Lamina propria

The loose connective tissue of the lamina propria forms the core of the villi. The remainder of the lamina propria, extending down to the muscularis mucosae, is compressed into thin sheets of highly vascularized connective tissue by the numerous tubular intestinal glands, or intestinal crypts. The lamina propria also is rich in lymphoid cells and contains occasional lymphoid nodules, which protect the intestinal lining from invasion by microorganisms. These lymphoid cells and lymph nodules belong to the gut-associated lymphoid tissue(GALT).

Intestinal crypts are simple tubular (or branched tubular) glands; they are composed of endocrine cells, surface absorptive-like columnar cells, goblet cells, regenerative cells, M cells, and Paneth cells.

A. Stem cells   The stem cell, of the small intestine are stem cells that undergo extensive proliferation to repopulate the epithelium of the crypts, mucosal surface, and villi. It has been suggested that five to seven days after the appearance of a new cell, that cell has progressed to the tip of the villus and has been exfoliated.

B. Paneth cells   Paneth cells produce the antibacterial agent lysozyme. Paneth cells are clearly distinguishable because of the presence of large, eosinophilic, apical secretory granules. These pyramid-shaped cells occupy the bottom of the intestinal crypts and manufacture the antibacterial agent lysozyme, defensive proteins (defensins). (Fig. 12-9)

Absorptive cells, endocrines cells and goblet cells also present on the lining of intestinal crypts.

iii. Muscularis mucosae

The muscularis mucosae of the small intestine is composed of an inner circular layer and an outer longitudinal layer of smooth muscle cells. Muscle fibers from the inner circular layer enter the villus and extend through its core to the tip of the connective tissue, as far as the basement membrane. During digestion, these muscle fibers rhythmically contract, shortening the villus so as to facilitate the absorption.

II. Submucosa

The submucosa of the small intestine is composed of dense, irregular fibroelastic connective tissue with a rich lymphatic and vascular supply; Meissner plexus may also be present here. The submucosa of the duodenum has the glands known as Brunner glands (duodenal glands), which produce a mucous, bicarbonate-rich fluid as well as urogastrone (human epidermal growth factor) (Fig. 12-10). This fluid helps neutralize the acidic chyme that enters the duodenum

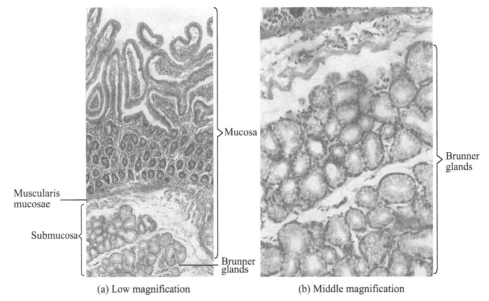

(a) Low magnification   (b) Middle magnification

Fig. 12-10   Sections of the duodenum

from the pyloric stomach.

III. Muscularis externa

The muscularis externa of the small intestine is composed of an inner circular layer and an outer longitudinal smooth muscle layer. Auerbach myenteric plexus is located between the two muscle layers. The muscularis externa is responsible for the peristaltic activity of the small intestine.

IV. Serosa

Except for the second and third parts of the duodenum which have fibrosa, the entire small intestine is invested by a serosa.

12.6   Large Intestine

The large intestine, is composed of the cecum, colon (ascending, transverse, descending, and sigmoid), rectum, and anus. It absorbs most of the water and ions from the chyme it receives from the small intestine and compacts the chyme into feces for elimination. The cecum and the colon are indistinguishable histologically and are discussed as a single entity called the colon.

12.6.1   Colon

The colon has no villi but is richly endowed with intestinal crypts that are similar in composition to those of the small intestine, except for the absence of Paneth cells. The number of goblet cells of its simple columnar epithelium increases from the cecum to the sigmoid colon, but throughout most of the colon, the surface absorptive cells are the most numerous cell type. Mucus on the surface of the lumen not only protects the mucosa of the colon but also facilitates the compaction of feces because it is the mucus that permits adherence of the solid wastes into a compact mass. Rapid mitotic activity of the regenerative cells replaces the epithelial lining of the crypts and of the mucosal surface every week (Fig. 12-11).

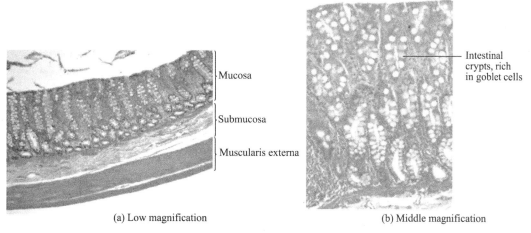

(a) Low magnification   (b) Middle magnification

Fig. 12-11   Section of the large intestine

The muscularis mucosae and submucosa of the colon resemble those of the small intestine. The muscularis externa is unusual in that the outer longitudinal layer is not of continuous thickness along the surface, but most of it is gathered into three narrow ribbons of muscle fascicles, known as taeniae coli. The serosa displays numerous fat-filled pouches, called appendices epiploicae.

12.6.2 Appendix

The histological appearance of the appendix resembles that of the colon, except that it is much smaller in diameter, has a richer supply of lymphoid elements, and contains many more endocrine cells in its intestinal crypts. Lymphoid tissue may extend between the muscularis externa and the luminal surface, replacing the submucosa and the mucosa. The appendix may become inflamed due to stagnation and impaction of the contents of the gut. This results in appendicitis. If the inflammation destroys the wall of the appendix, it spreads into the peritoneal cavity. As a result, microorganisms from the gut enter a large potential space where they can readily multiply; this may be fatal. (Fig. 12-12)

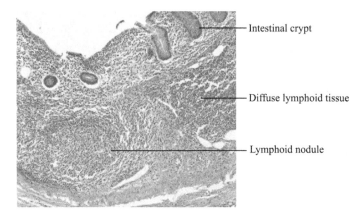

— Intestinal crypt

— Diffuse lymphoid tissue

— Lymphoid nodule

Fig. 12-12　Section of the appendix

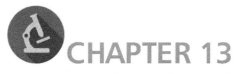

CHAPTER 13
DIGESTIVE GLANDS

T he digestive glands include the major salivary glands associated with the oral cavity (parotid, submandibular, and sublingual glands), the pancreas, and the liver and gallbladder. Each of these glands has functions aiding the digestive process, and their secretory products are delivered to the lumen of the alimentary tract by a system of ducts.

13.1　Major Salivary Glands

Saliva produced by salivary glands facilitates the process of tasting food, initiates its digestion, and permits its deglutition (swallowing). These glands also protect the body by secreting the antibacterial agents, lysozyme and lactoferrin as well as the secretory immunoglobulin IgA.

13.1.1　Generals of salivary glands

There are three pairs of major salivary glands: parotid, sublingual, and submandibular. They are branched tubuloacinar glands whose connective tissue capsule provides septa that subdivide the glands into lobes and lobules. Each of the major salivary glands has a secretory and a duct portion. (Fig. 13-1)

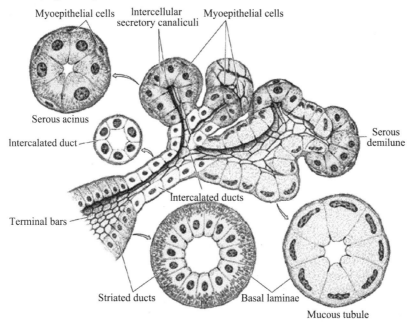

Fig. 13-1　Diagram of salivary glands

I. Secretory portions

The secretory portions of salivary glands are composed of serous and/or mucous secretory cells arranged in acini or tubules. Two types of secretory cell, serous and mucous cells, are present in the acini and, respectively, they produce a watery secretion containing proteins which function as enzymes and a viscous mucus in which large carbohydrate complexes are major components. In addition, myoepithelial cells wrap around the acini and their contractions help to expel the secretions.

- ◆ Serous Acini: Serous acini are composed of serous cells. Serous cells resemble truncated pyramids and have single, round, basally located nuclei, a well-developed rough endoplasmic reticulum, and Golgi complex, and abundant apically situated secretory granules rich in salivary amylase, which is an enzyme that initiates the digestion of complex carbohydrates.

- ◆ Mucous Acini: Mucous acini consist of mucous cells. Mucous cells are similar in shape to the serous cells. Their nuclei are also basally located but are flattened. Comparing with the serous cells, the mucous cells have fewer mitochondria, a less extensive RER, and a considerably greater Golgi apparatus, indicative of the greater carbohydrate component of their secretory product. The apical region of the cytoplasm is occupied by abundant secretory granules housing mucinogen, which, when released into the ducts of the gland, becomes hydrated and is known as mucin. When mucin contacts and is intermixed with substances present in the oral cavity, it becomes known as mucus.

- ◆ Mixed Acini: Mixed acini are composed of both serous and mucus cells.

II. Duct portions

The ducts of major salivary glands are highly branched and range from very small intercalated ducts to very large principal ducts. The smallest branches of the system of ducts are the intercalated ducts, to which the secretory acini are attached. These small ducts are composed of a single layer of low cuboidal cells and possess some myoepithelial cells.

Several intercalated ducts merge with each other to form striated ducts, composed of a single layer of cuboidal to low columnar cells. The basolateral cell membranes of these cells have sodium adenosine triphosphatase (Na^+-ATPase) that pump sodium out of the cell into the connective tissue, thus conserving these ions and reducing the tonicity of saliva.

Striated ducts join with each other, forming intralobular ducts of increasing caliber, which are surrounded by more abundant connective tissue elements. Interlobular ducts form intralobar and interlobar ducts. The terminal (principal) duct of the gland delivers saliva into the oral cavity.

III. Salivon

The acinus, intercalated duct, and striated duct together constitute the salivon, the functional unit of a salivary gland.

13.1.2 Parotid gland

The parotid glands are the largest of the salivary glands and each parotid gland is located close to an ear. Serous acini form the majority of the parenchyma of the parotid glands. Adipose cells appear in the parotid glands with age. Many small ducts are distributed throughout the parenchyma of parotid glands and they are lined by epithelial cells which stain readily with eosin. (Fig. 13-2)

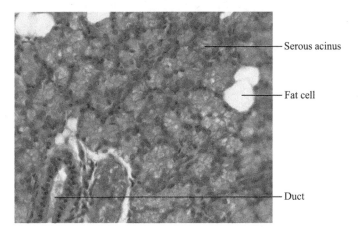

Fig. 13-2   Section of the parotid gland

The saliva produced by the parotid gland has high levels of the enzyme salivary amylase (ptyalin) and secretory IgA. Salivary amylase is responsible for digestion of most of the starch in food, and secretory IgA inactivates antigens located in the oral cavity.

13.1.3   Submandibular glands

The submandibular glands lie beneath the mandible on each side, wrapped around the muscle which supports the tongue. Each gland drains to the undersurface of the tongue. Mucous acini are a prominent feature of submandibular glands, but serous cells are also present. The arrangement of the serous and mucous gland cells together in some acini is such that these are described as mucous glands with serous demilunes. (Fig. 13-3)

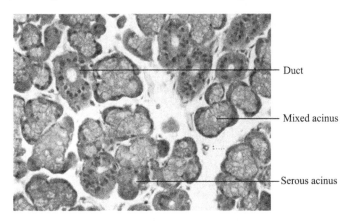

Fig. 13-3   Section of the submandibular gland

13.1.4   Sublingual glands

The sublingual glands are the smallest of the salivary glands. Mucous gland cells are predominant in sublingual glands and the ducts open directly into the floor of the oral cavity, rather than via a single duct system. (Fig. 13-4)

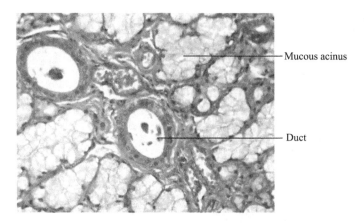

— Mucous acinus

— Duct

Fig. 13-4　Section of the sublingual gland

13.2　Pancreas

The pancreas is both an exocrine gland that produces digestive juices and an endocrine gland that manufactures hormones. The pancreas manufactures a bicarbonate-rich fluid that buffers the acid chyme in the duodenum and produces enzymes necessary for the digestion of fats, proteins, and carbohydrates. In addition, the islets of Langerhans of the pancreas synthesize and release endocrine hormones, including insulin, glucagon, somatostatin, gastrin, and pancreatic polypeptide. (Fig. 13-5)

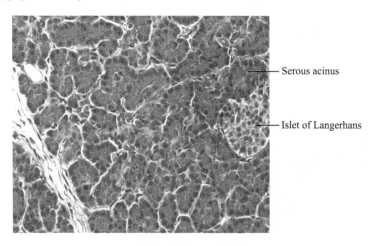

— Serous acinus

— Islet of Langerhans

Fig. 13-5　Section of the pancreas

13.2.1　Exocrine pancreas

The exocrine pancreas is a compound tubuloacinar gland that produces the pancreatic juice containing digestive proenzymes. Serous acinar cells form a round to oval acinus. The acinar cells manufacture, store, and release a large number of enzymes: including trypsinogen, pancreatic amylase, lipase, cholesterol esterase, ribonuclease (RNase), deoxyribonuclease (DNase) and elastase which will participate in the digestion of nutrients of the food in duodenum. The enzymes are stored in zymogen granules in the apical portions of the serous cells; the nucleus and rough endoplasmic reticulum are in the basal portions of the cells. The cells also manufacture trypsin inhibitor, a protein that protects the cell from accidental intracellular activation of trypsin as well as its activation in the pancreatic duct.

The lumen of the acinus is occupied by several centroacinar cells, the beginning of the duct system of the pancreas. The centroacinar cells are pale and low cuboidal. The duct system of the pancreas begins within the center of the acinus with the terminus of the intercalated ducts. Ducts join together within the lobules and eventually all join and form a single pancreatic duct. The pancreatic duct joins the bile duct and bile and pancreatic juices drain into the duodenum. The centroacinar cells and intercalated ducts manufacture a serous, alkaline fluid, which neutralizes and buffers the acid chyme that enters the duodenum from the pyloric stomach.

13.2.2 Endocrine pancreas

The endocrine pancreas is composed of spherical aggregates of cells, known as islets of Langerhans, scattering among the acini. Each islet of Langerhans is a richly vascularized. The approximately 1 to 2 million islets are distributed throughout the human pancreas. Five types of cells compose the parenchyma of each islet, as follows:

I. Alpha (α) cells (A-cells)

These cells take up 20% islet of Langerhans in cell number, located at the periphery. They secrete glucagon, which raise blood glucose level.

II. Beta (β) cells (B-cells)

These cells take up 70%, located in the central portion. They secrete insulin lowering blood glucose level. Damage of B-cells induces diabetes.

III. Delta (δ) cells (D-cells)

These cells take up 5%, scattering between A-cells or B-cells. They secrete somatostatin which inhibits the release of insulin and glucagon.

IV. PP cells

These cells just are in a small amount, which produce pancreatic polypeptide. This hormone inhibits the exocrine secretions of the pancreas and the release of bile from the gallbladder. It also stimulates the release of enzymes by the gastric chief cells while depressing the release of HCl by the parietal cells of the stomach.

V. G cells

G cells are the few scatted cells in the islet of Langerhans. Gastrin, released by G cells, stimulates gastric release of HCl, gastric motility and emptying, and the rate of cell division in gastric regenerative cells.

13.3 Liver

The liver, is the largest gland in the body. It is located in the upper right of the abdominal cavity. Similar to the pancreas, the liver has both endocrine and exocrine functions; unlike the pancreas, however, the same cell (the hepatocyte) in the liver is responsible for the formation of the liver's exocrine secretion, bile, and its numerous endocrine products.

Bile is required for proper absorption of lipids, whereas many of the liver's endocrine functions are essential for life. These functions include metabolism of proteins, lipids, and carbohydrates; synthesis of blood proteins and coagulation factors; manufacture of vitamins; and detoxification of blood-borne toxins.

The gallbladder concentrates bile and stores it until its release into the lumen of the duodenum.

Structurally, the parenchyma of liver is composed of liver hepatic lobules.

13.3.1　Hepatic lobule

The hexagon-shape hepatic lobule is the structural and the functional unit of liver, mainly composed of hepatocytes, which are arranged in plates, radiating from the central vein toward the periphery of the lobule. These lobules are clearly demarcated by slender connective tissue elements in animals such as the pig. However, because of the scarcity of connective tissue and the closely paced arrangement of the lobules in humans, the boundaries of the classical lobules can only be approximated. (Fig. 13-6)

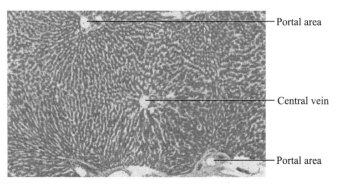

(a) Section of the liver (low magnification)

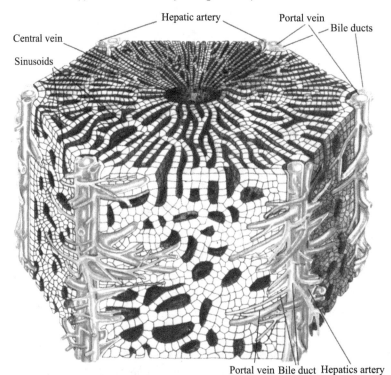

(b) Diagram of a hepatic lobule

Fig. 13-6　Hepatic lobule

I. Hepatocyte and hepatic plates

The hepatocytes, the cells of the main parenchymal tissue of the liver, make up 70% ~ 85% of the total liver cells. The hepatocytes are 5-to 12-sided polygonal cells, approximately 20 to 30 μm in diameter, that are closely packed together to form anastomosing plates of liver cells, hepatic plates, which are separated by vascular channels (sinusoids), an arrangement supported by a reticulin (collagen type Ⅲ) network.

Hepatocytes display an eosinophilic cytoplasm, reflecting numerous mitochondria, and basophilic stippling due to large amounts of rough endoplasmic reticulum and free ribosomes. Brown lipofuscin granules are also observed (with increasing age) together with irregular unstained areas of cytoplasm; these correspond to cytoplasmic glycogen and lipid stores removed during histological preparation. Hepatocyte nuclei are round with dispersed chromatin and prominent nucleoli. Binucleate or even tetranucleate cells are observed. The average life span of the hepatocyte is five months; and they are able to regenerate.

The hepatocytes are involved in protein synthesis and storage; transformation of carbohydrates; synthesis of cholesterol, bile salts and phospholipids; detoxification, modification, and excretion of exogenous and endogenous substances; and initiation of formation and secretion of bile. (Fig. 13-7)

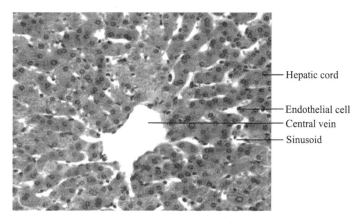

Hepatic cord

Endothelial cell
Central vein
Sinusoid

Fig. 13-7   Section of the liver(high magnification)

II. Hepatic sinusoids

Between the hepatic plates, large vascular spaces are known as hepatic sinusoids, and the blood flowing in these wide vessels, lined by endothelial cells. Often, the cells of this endothelial lining do not make contact with each other, leaving gaps of up to 0.5 μm between them. The sinusoidal lining cells also have fenestrae that are present in clusters. Thus, particulate matter less than 0.5 μm in diameter may leave the lumen of the sinusoid.

Resident macrophages, known as Kupffer cells, have processes and are intermingled with the sinusoidal lining cells of the sinusoids and they phagocytose effete red cells and microorganisms if present in the blood. (Fig. 13-8)

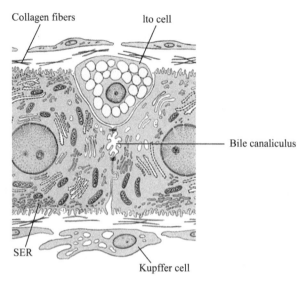

Fig. 13-8   Diagram of space of Disse

III. Space of Disse

The thin gaps between the hepatocytes and their adjacent sinusoid-lining epithelial cells are known as space of Disse. The space contains the blood plasma and delicate fibers that support the sinusoids. Microvilli of hepatocytes extend into this space, allowing proteins and other plasma components from the sinusoids to be absorbed by the hepatocytes. Fenestration and discontinuity of the endothelium, as well as its basement membrane, facilitates this transport. This space may be obliterated in liver disease, leading to decreased uptake by hepatocytes of nutrients and wastes such as bilirubin. (Fig. 13-8)

The space also contains the cells of Ito, which store fat or fat soluble vitamins (including vitamin A). A variety of infections that cause inflammation can result in the cells transforming into myofibroblasts, resulting in collagen production, fibrosis, and cirrhosis.

IV. Bile canaliculi

Bile canaliculus is a thin channel between adjacent hepatocytes that collects bile secreted by hepatocytes (Fig. 13-8). The canaliculi is protected by the formation of tight junctions between adjoining liver cells, isolating these channels from the remaining extracellular space. Short microvilli project from the hepatocyte into the bile canaliculi, thus increasing the surface areas through which bile can be secreted. The bile canaliculi receive bile secreted by hepatocytes. The direction of flow in bile canaliculi is opposite to the blood flow in sinusoids. Namely from the center of the hepatic lobules to the periphery, the canaliculus join together and drain into the interlobular bile ducts at the portal area.

13.3.2   Portal area

Where three hepatic lobules are in contact with each other, the connective tissue elements are increased, and these regions are known as portal areas. In addition to lymph vessels, portal areas house the following three structures (portal triads), the branches of the hepatic arteries, the hepatic portal veins and the interlobular bile ducts. (Fig. 13-9)

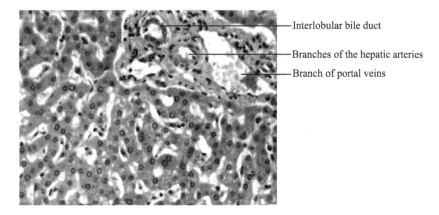

Fig. 13-9   **Section of the liver showing the portal area**

13.3.3 Blood supply

The liver has a dual blood supply, receiving oxygenated blood from the left and right hepatic arteries (~25%) and hemoglobin-rich blood from the spleen as well as nutrient-rich blood from the digestive tract via the portal vein (~75%). Both vessels enter the liver at the porta hepatis. The branches of the hepatic arteries and the portal vein at the portal areas then pass into liver sinusoids. As blood enters the sinusoids, its flow slows considerably, and it slowly percolates into the central veins, which join together and leave the liver as the hepatic vein. (Fig. 13-10)

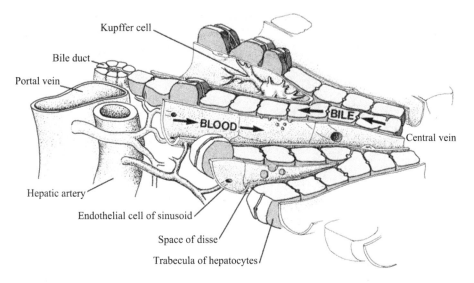

Fig. 13-10   **Blood supply and route of bile juice of hepatic lobule**

13.3.4 Models of the liver organization

There are three models of the liver organizations: the classic lobule, the portal lobule, and liver acinus models, depending upon their functional significance.

I . Classic lobule model

This model, as described above, emphasizes the endocrine function. It is based on the arrangement of the branches of the portal vein and hepatic artery (the path of blood flow as it perfuses the hepatocytes). The boundaries of the classic lobules are defined by connective tissue septa from the capsule.

II. Portal lobule model

The portal lobule model emphasizes the exocrine function of the liver, namely bile secretion. The portal bile duct is at the center. Its outer margins are imaginary lines drawn between three central veins that are closest to that portal triad.

III. Liver acinus model

This model has at its center the blood supply (portal and arterial) to the liver parenchyma, rather than its venous drainage; emphasizes oxygen and nutrient gradient. This model describes the smallest functional unit in the liver parenchyma. The ovoid hepatic acinus model centers on the portal triad (trunk) and projects acinar sinusoids (branches) to terminal hepatic veins. Cells in the liver acinus are arranged into three concentric, elliptical zones. Zone I cells, the closest to distributing arteries and veins, are the first to be affected by or to alter the incoming blood and receive both nutrients and toxins. If circulation is impaired, they are the last to die and the first to regenerate. (Fig. 13-11)

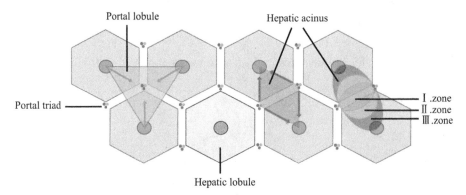

Fig. 13-11　Three models of the liver organizations

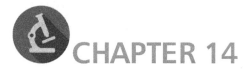

CHAPTER 14
ENDOCRINE SYSTEM

The endocrine system comprises cells which synthesise hormones and secrete them into blood vessels. Hormones are carried by the vascular circulation around the body where they interact with target cells. Hormones achieve their specific action by interacting with receptor molecules expressed by the target cells in various tissues and organs. In general, hormones are involved in regulating metabolic activities in cells in many organs and tissues of the body, many of which are important in controlling homeostasis.

All endocrine glands and endocrine cells are well vascularized, and the capillaries in endocrine glands are fenestrated and most hormones are secreted directly into them. Hormones are of two types: nitrogen-containing hormones and steroid hormones; and accordingly, endocrine cells are classified into two types according to chemical nature of hormones released.

◆ Nitrogen-containing hormone-secreting cells: They are found in thyroid, parathyroids, adrenal medulla, pituitary and pineal glands, etc. The cells contain RER, Golgi complex and membrane bound secretory granules. Hormones are secreted by exocytosis and the receptors of hormones are located in the cell membranes.

◆ Steroid hormone-secreting cells: They are found only in adrenal cortex and gonads. The cells contain abundant SER, mitochondria with tubular cristae (Fig. 14-1) and lipid droplets. Hormones are secreted by diffusion and the receptors of hormones are located in the nucleuses of the cells.

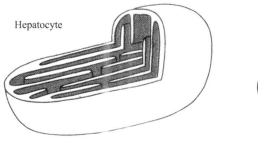

Hepatocyte

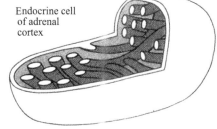

Endocrine cell of adrenal cortex

(a) Regular mitochondria   (b) Mitochondria with tubular cristae

Fig. 14-1   Two types of mitochondria

The endocrine organs comprise the pituitary gland, thyroid gland, parathyroid glands, adrenal glands and the pineal gland.

14.1 Thyroid Gland

The thyroid gland lies anterior to the lower part of the larynx and upper trachea. It comprises two lobes joined by the isthmus.

The parenchyma of thyroid consists of spherical follicles of various sizes whose total number may exceed 20 million. Follicle cavities are filled with gelatinous colloid made of thyroglobulin, the temporary storage form and precursor to main thyroid hormones before release. (Fig. 14-2)

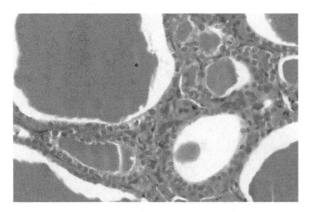

Fig. 14-2　Section of the thyroid gland
* Colloid in the follicle of thyroid

Follicles of thyroid are lined by simple cuboidal epithelium, which consists of follicular cells and parafollicular cells. In the cavity of follicle, present the homogeneous, acidophilic, gelatinous substance, known as colloid, whose chemical composition is iodinated thyroglobulin. The height of the epithelium varies with function: usually low cuboidal in an underactive gland and high in an overactive one. A large network of fenestrated capillaries is in delicate reticular connective tissue between follicles.

I . Follicular cells

These cells synthesize and release thyroid hormones. The process is as following. Amino acids are taken up from the bloodstream at the base of follicular cells. The pre-thyroglobulin is synthesized on the rough endoplasmic reticulum (RER), followed by glycosylation in the RER and Golgi apparatus, and packaging in vesicles. Fusion of vesicles with apical plasma membrane leads to exocytosis of thyroglobulin into follicle cavity. Meanwhile, uptake of circulating iodide at the cell basal membrane is followed by oxidation by peroxidase and transfer to cell apices. Enzymes in apical microvilli that project into colloid catalyze iodination of tyrosine residues in thyroglobulin. Stimulation by TSH causes follicular cells to pinocytose portions of colloid and form vesicles containing iodinated thyroglobulin. They fuse with lysosomes that cleave thyroglobulin. Resultant T3 (triiodothyronine) and T4 (thyroxine) are released into the bloodstream.

T3 and T4 increase oxygen consumption and metabolic rates of most body tissues and are essential for normal growth, maturation, and mental activity. (Fig. 14-3)

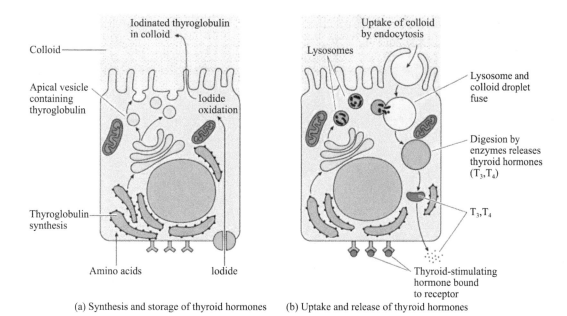

(a) Synthesis and storage of thyroid hormones   (b) Uptake and release of thyroid hormones

Fig. 14-3   Diagram of the synthesis and release of thyroid hormones

II. Parafollicular cells

Small numbers of larger and paler parafollicular cells lie, as single cells or small groups, between the basement membrane of the follicles and follicular cells, or in an interfollicular position. These cells secrete calcitonin, which lowers blood calcium levels and counterbalances actions of parathyroid hormone. Hard to see in routine histologic sections, they are best revealed by immunocytochemical methods or silver staining. (Fig. 14-4)

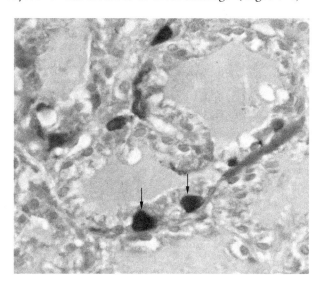

Fig. 14-4   Section of the thyroid gland, silver-stained, showing the parafollicular cells(arrows)

14.2   Parathyroid Glands

The parathyroid glands are small paired structures on the posterior surface of the thyroid gland. Humans usually have four parathyroid glands. There are two major parenchymal cell types, chief cells and oxyphil cells. (Fig. 14-5)

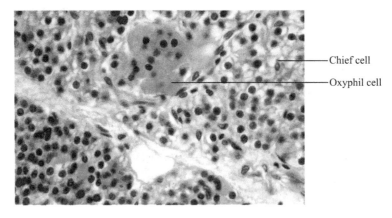
Chief cell
Oxyphil cell

Fig. 14-5   Section of the parathyroid gland

I . Chief cells

Chief cells are relatively small and secrete parathyroid hormone (PTH). PTH assists in maintenance of calcium levels in the blood. Low levels of calcium in blood stimulate the secretion of PTH. Calcitonin and PTH have opposite effects and together affect the mineralization of bone via the activity of osteoclasts.

II . Oxyphil Cells

Oxyphil cells are larger and stain with dyes such as eosin and their role is not known.

14.3   Adrenal Gland

The paired adrenal glands lie on the superior pole of each kidney and are embedded in adipose tissue. They are invested by the connective tissue capsule. The parenchyma of the gland is divided into two regions: an outer portion known as cortex and an inner portion called medulla. (Fig. 14-6)

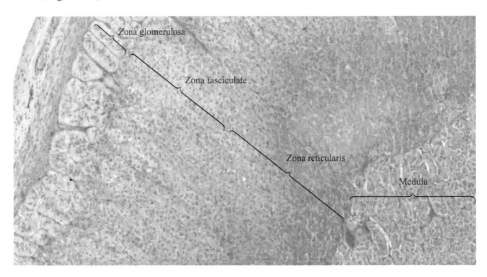
Zona glomerulosa
Zona fasciculate
Zona reticularis
Medula

Fig. 14-6   Section of the adrenal gland

14.3.1   Cortex

The cortex contains parenchymal cells that synthesize and secrete several steroid hormones without storing them. Three concentric zones characterize the cortex: zona glomerulosa, zona fasciculate and zona reticularis.

I . Zona glomerulosa

The zona glomerulosa, just under the capsule, represents 10% ~15% of the cortex. The small columnar cells composing this zone are arranged in clusters. The parenchymal cells produce mineralocorticoids, mainly aldosterone. Synthesis of these hormones is stimulated by renin-angiotensin system. The mineralocorticoid hormones function in controlling fluid and electrolyte balance in the body by affecting the function of the renal tubules, specifically the distal convoluted tubules (see Chapter 15).

II . Zona fasciculata

The middle zone of the medulla is zona fasciculata, forming up to 70% ~ 80% of the cortex, and consists mainly of radially oriented cords of polyhedral cells. The cells in this layer are larger than the cells of the zona glomerulosa and contain many lipid droplets. The sinusoidal capillaries are arranged longitudinally between the columns of cells. Cells of the zona fasciculata synthesize and secrete the glucocorticoid hormones, cortisol and corticosterone. The synthesis of these hormones is stimulated by ACTH. Glucocorticoids function in the control of carbohydrate, fat, and protein metabolism. These hormones also suppress the immune response.

III. Zona reticularis

It makes up 5% ~10% of the cortex. Its smaller, more acidophilic parenchymal cells are arranged as an anastomosing network of short cords with intervening sinusoidal capillaries. These cells synthesize androgens. Additionally, cells of the zona reticularis may synthesize and secrete small amounts of glucocorticoids. The secretion of these hormones is stimulated by ACTH.

14.3.2   Medulla

The medulla consists of chromaffin cells and numerous capillaries.

Chromaffin cells are large, arranged in clusters or short cords; they contain granules that stain intensely with chromic salts. The granules can be stained deep brown when exposed to chromaffin salts. Chromaffin cells produce the catecholamines (epinephrine and norepinephrine) and are surrounded by fenestrated capillaries. They are modified postganglionic sympathetic neurons that produce two classes of catecholamines: epinephrine and norepinephrine. Catecholamines cause general physiological changes that prepare the body for physical activity (fight-or-flight response). Some typical effects are increases in heart rate, blood pressure, blood glucose levels, and a general reaction of the sympathetic nervous system.

The secretion of the chromaffin cells is stimulated by preganglionic sympathetic (cholinergic) splanchnic nerves.

14.4   Pituitary Gland

The pituitary gland (hypophysis) lies in the midline in a depression of the sphenoid bone, the sella turcica. It has two major subdivisions: the adenohypophysis and the neurohypophysis. (Fig. 14-7)

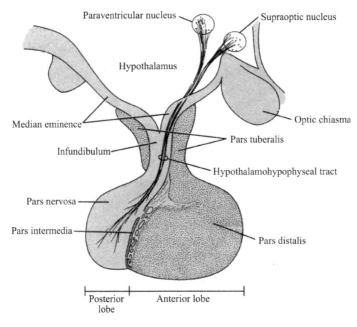

Fig. 14-7   Diagram of pituitary gland

14.4.1 Adenohypophysis

The adenohypophysis consists of three parts, the pars distalis (anterior lobe), the pars intermedia and the pars tuberalis.

I. Pars distalis

The glandular cells of the pars distalis are of three types: acidophils, basophils and chromophobes. In routine HE preparations, the acidophils have acidophilic granules in cytoplasm, whereas, the basophils have basophilic granules. (Fig. 14-8)

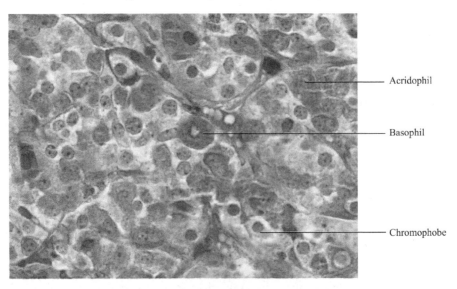

Fig. 14-8   Section of the pituitary gland showing the pars distalis

ⅰ. Acidophils

The acidophils take up about 40% total glandular cells in the pars distalis. With EM and immunohistochemical techniques, there are two varieties of the acidophils: somatotrophs and mammotrophs (lactotrophs).

- ◆ Somatotrophs: These cells produce growth hormone (GH). GH is important in stimulating growth, particularly in bones.
- ◆ mammotrophs (lactotrophs): These cells produce prolactin (PL). PL has a major effect on milk production by the mammary glands and is also known as mammotrophin.

ⅱ. Basophils

The basophils take up about 10% total glandular cells of the pars distalis and with EM and immunohistochemical techniques, three types of the basophils are shown: thyrotrophs, corticotrophs and gonadotrophs.

- ◆ Thyrotrophs: Thyrotrophs secrete thyrotropin or thyroid stimulating hormone (TSH), which stimulates growth of thyroid follicles and synthesis and release of thyroid hormones.
- ◆ Corticotrophs: Corticotrophs secrete adrenocorticotrophic hormone (ACTH), which stimulates secretion of glucocorticoids from zona fasciculata and reticularis of adrenal cortex.
- ◆ Gonadotrophs: Gonadotrophs secrete follicle-stimulating hormone (FSH) and luteinizing hormone (LH). FSH promotes ovarian follicle development in females and spermatogenesis in males. LH promotes ovulation and development of the corpus luteum in female. In male LH stimulates androgen secretion by Leydig cells.

ⅲ. Chromophobes

The chromophobes take up about 50% total glandular cells of the pars distalis. These cells are clusters of small cells without distinct boundaries and pale stained. Few secretory granules indicates that they are undifferentiated precursor cells or degranulated chromophils.

Ⅱ. Pars intermedia

The pars intermedia is composed of chromophobes and basophil cells arranged either in cords or in colloid-containing follicles. These cells secrete melanocyte stimulating hormone (MSH) which promotes the production of melanin in melanocytess.

Ⅲ. Pars tuberalis

The pars tuberalis surrounds the infundibulum, and the cells arranged in cords separated by sinusoids. Most cells secrete FSH and LH in humans.

Ⅳ. Relationship between pars distalis and hypothalamus

Activities of the cells in the pars distalis are controlled by hypothalamic neuroendocrine neurons that produce peptide releasing hormones and inhibitory hormones, which are transported to the pars distalis through the hypophyseal portal system. Hypophyseal portal system includes:

- ◆ The primary capillary plexus in the stalk and median eminence, formed by superior hypophyseal arteries.
- ◆ The hypophyseal portal venules from the primary plexus in pars tuberalis.
- ◆ The secondary capillary plexus in pars distalis, formed from the portal venules.

This portal system is critical for the control of the adenohypophysis by neurosecretions from hypothalamic neurons that convey releasing and inhibiting hormones to the primary plexus. (Fig. 14-9)

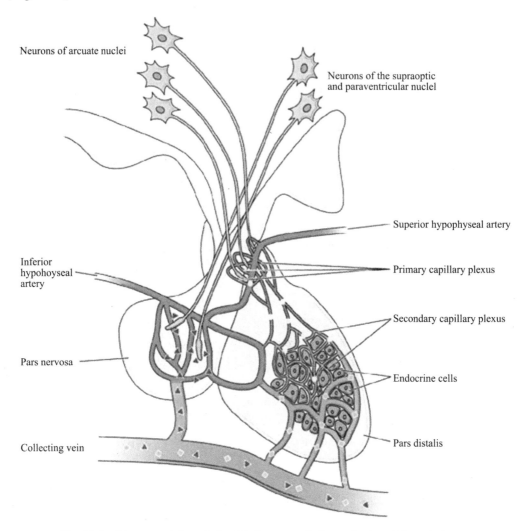

Neurons of arcuate nuclei

Neurons of the supraoptic and paraventricular nuclei

Superior hypophyseal artery

Inferior hypohoyseal artery

Primary capillary plexus

Secondary capillary plexus

Endocrine cells

Pars nervosa

Collecting vein

Pars distalis

Fig. 14-9   Diagram of the relationship between pituitary gland and hypothalamus

14.4.2   Neurohypophysis

The neurohypophysis is situated at the posterior of the pituitary gland. It develops from a downgrowth of the hypothalamus and thus is composed of nerve tissue. The neurohypophysis is divided into the median eminence, the infundibulum (continuation of the hypothalamus), and the pars nervosa.

Pars nervosa contains large numbers of unmyelinated nerve fibers, sinusoids and unmyelinated nerve fibers. The nerve fibers contain neurosecretory granules, which often accumulate in the axons. They originate from neurons of hypothalamic supraoptic and paraventricular nuclei, which produce vasopressin (antidiuretic hormone, ADH) and oxytocin. These dilated expansions of the axons contain aggregates of neurosecretory material, which are stored before release, forming Herring bodies. By light microscopy, these bodies appear as amorphous, lightly eosinophilic amorphous areas in close contact with capillaries. (Fig. 14-10)

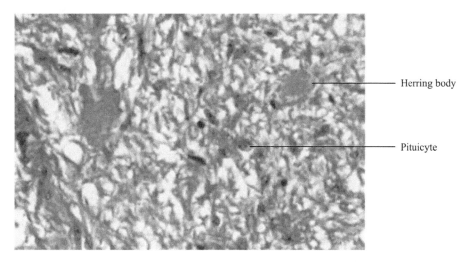

Herring body

Pituicyte

Fig. 14-10   Section of the pituitary gland showing the pars nervosa

The two hormones released in pars nervosa are:
- Vasopressin: It stimulates water resorption in kidneys and contraction of vascular smooth muscle.
- Oxytocin: It promotes contraction of uterine smooth muscle during parturition and contraction of myoepithelial cells in mammary glands during lactation.

The neuroglial cells in pars nervosa are known as pituicytes, which are irregular shaped and with short processes. These cells contain lipid droplets and pigment granules in their cytoplasm.

Median eminence contains neurons that secrete the hypothalamic releasing hormones which regulate the secretory activity of cells in the pars distalis of the pituitary. Infundibulum is the continuation of the hypothalamus.

An overview of the regulations of hypothalamus and pituitary gland on the target tissues is shown in Fig. 14-11.

14.5   Pineal Body

The pineal body is located in the epithalamus, tucked in a groove where the two halves of the thalamus join. It is a small endocrine gland, with the shape like a pine cone. It consists of pinealocytes, astrocytes and unmyelinated nerve fibers. Pinealocytes are slightly basophilic, with secretory granules and long processes. Pinealocytes produce, mainly at night, melatonin that regulates circadian rhythm.

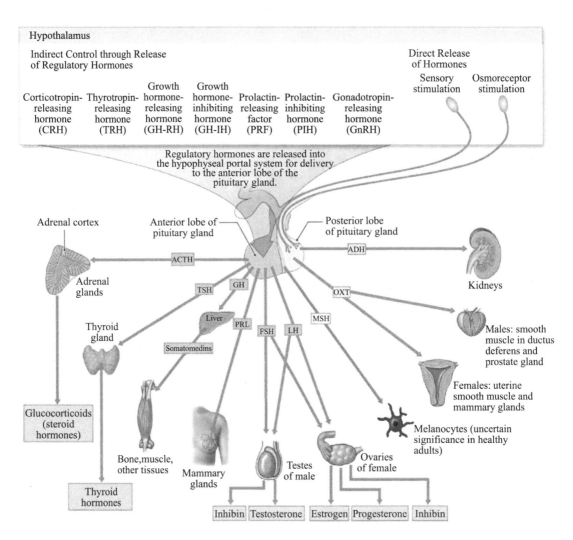

Fig. 14-11 An overview of the regulations of hypothalamus and pituitary gland on the target tissues in body

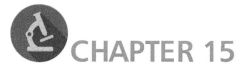

CHAPTER 15
THE URINARY SYSTEM

The urinary system consists of paired kidneys and the urinary tract. The urinary tract which comprises paired ureters, a urinary bladder and a urethra. The urinary system removes toxic byproducts of metabolism from the bloodstream by forming urine. These actions are performed by the two kidneys, which not only remove the toxins, but also conserve salts, glucose, proteins, and water as well as additional materials essential for proper health. Because of these eliminating and conserving functions, the kidneys also help regulate blood pressure, hematopoiesis and the acid base balance of the body. Urine is delivered from the kidneys into the two ureters, stored in the urinary bladder and emptied via the urethra to outside the body.

15.1 Kidney

The kidneys are large bean-shaped organs situated on the posterior abdominal wall. The kidney is invested by a thin capsule, consisting of dense irregular collagenous connective tissue. The kidney has a concave region, known as the hilum, where the ureter, renal vein, renal artery, and lymph vessels enter or exit. The ureter is expanded at this region, forming the renal pelvis. A fat-filled extension of the hilum deeper into the kidney is called the renal sinus. (Fig. 15-1)

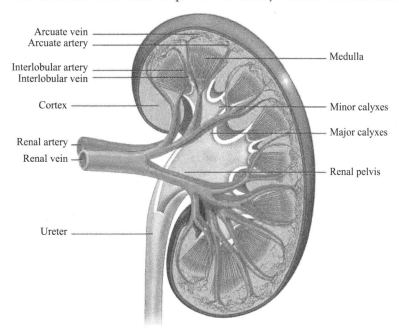

Fig. 15-1 Diagram of gross anatomy of kidney

15.1.1 Gross structure

A section of the kidney shows that it is separated into a cortex and a medulla. The cortical region appears dark brown in fresh, whereas the medulla contains 6 ~ 12 discrete, pyramid-shaped, pale renal pyramids. From the base of each pyramid, several medullary rays are given rise toward the cortex, whereas its apex, known as the renal papilla, points toward the hilum. The cortical regions between the two adjacent medullary rays are known as the cortical labyrinth. The apex of the renal pyramid is surrounded by a cup-like space, the minor calyx, which, joining two or three neighboring minor calyces, forms a major calyx. The three or four major calyces empty into the renal pelvis, the expanded continuation of the proximal portion of the ureter. Neighboring pyramids are separated from each other by the structure resembling the cortex, the cortical columns.

The portion of the cortex overlying the base of each pyramid is known as a cortical arch. A renal pyramid, with its associated cortical arch and cortical columns, represents a lobe of the kidney. Each medullary ray with part of the cortical labyrinth surrounding it is considered a kidney lobule (Fig. 15-1, Fig. 15-2).

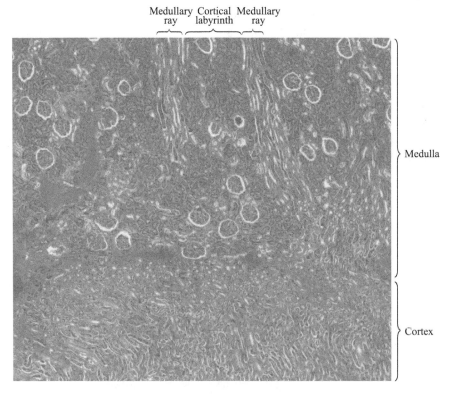

Fig. 15-2　Section of the kidney (low magnification)

15.1.2 Histology of kidney

The parenchyma of the kidney consists of two parts, the nephron and the collecting tubule (Fig. 15-3). There are about a million nephrons in each kidney in humans. A nephron consists of a renal corpuscle, which filters blood. The uriniferous tubule, which consists of the renal tubule together with the collecting tubule, is attached to the renal corpuscle, drains and modifies the filtrate. Eventually, the modified filtrate becomes urine and drains, via the renal pelvis, into the ureter.

The arrangement of the histological structure of kidney is shown in Tab. 15-1.

Tab. 15-1   Histological components of kidney

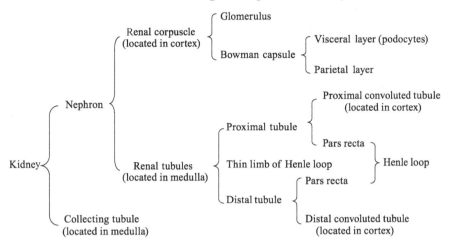

I. Nephron

The nephron is composed of the renal corpuscle and the renal tubules. There are two types of nephrons, depending on the location of their renal corpuscles and the length of their Henle loop: superficial and juxtamedullary. The former presents at the superficial cortical region and the latter close to the medullar. Henle loops of the former are quite short, by contrast, the Henle loops of juxtamedullary nephrons extend deep into the medulla and play a significant role in the concentration of the urine, though they constitute only 15% of all nephrons (Fig. 15-3).

i. Renal corpuscle

The renal corpuscle is composed of a tuft the renal glomerulus, surrounded by Bowman capsule (Fig. 15-4, Fig. 15-5). The renal corpuscle has two poles: the region where the vessels enter and exit Bowman capsule is the vascular pole, whereas the region close to the proximal tubule, is the urinary pole.

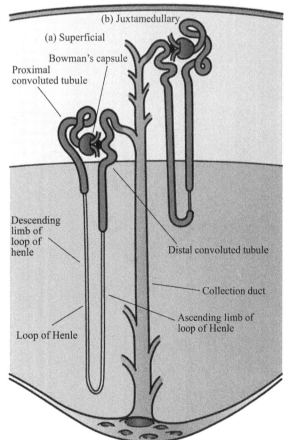

Fig. 15-3   Diagram of two types of nephrons

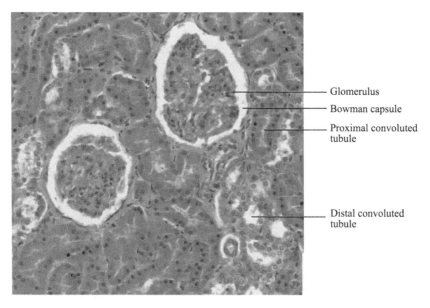

Fig. 15-4 Section of the kidney showing the cortex

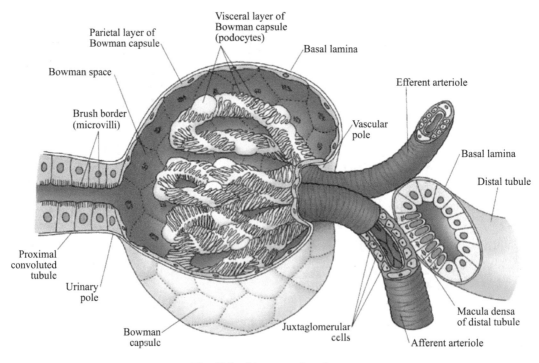

Fig. 15-5 Diagram of nephron

A. Glomerulus   The glomerulus is a network of capillaries from the afferent arteriole. It is located at the beginning of a nephron, invested by Bowman capsule. It serves as the first stage in the filtering process of the blood in its formation of urine.

The glomerulus receives its blood supply from an afferent arteriole. Unlike most other capillary beds, the glomerulus drains into an efferent arteriole rather than a venule. The resistance of these arterioles results in high pressure within the glomerulus, facilitating the process of filtration, where fluids and soluble materials in the blood are forced out of the capillaries and into Bowman capsule.

The glomerulus is the fenestrated capillaries and the fenestrae of the walls of the capillaries are usually not covered by a diaphragm. The pores are large, ranging between 70 ~ 90 nm in diameter; hence, these capillaries act as a barrier only to formed elements of the blood and to macromolecules whose effective diameter exceeds the size of the fenestrae (e. g. albumin). Investing the endothelial cells of the glomerulus is a basal lamina. (Fig. 15-5, Fig. 15-6)

The capillaries within the glomerulus are connected and supported by the thin membrane, the mesangial membrane, which has a specialized cell type known as the intraglomerular mesangial cells. The functions of intraglomerular mesangial cells are:

- ◆ phagocytose the Ab-Ag complex that may be deposited in the glomerular basal lamina and function in renewal of the basal lamina to maintain the proper permeability of the filtration barrier;
- ◆ be contractile to regulate the diameter of the capillaries so as to regulate the glomerular perfusion flow;
- ◆ synthesize various cytokines, such as interleukin-1, endothelins, etc;
- ◆ provide physical support to the capillaries of the glomerulus.

B. Bowman capsule   Bowman capsule is a two-layered cup-like sack that holds the glomerulus. Its two layers are the inner visceral layer and the outer parietal layer, and between the two layers is Bowman space.

- ◆ Visceral layer: The visceral layer of Bowman capsule is composed of the podocytes. These large cells bear numerous long, tentacle-like extensions, the primary processes. Each primary process bears many secondary processes, known as the pedicels, parallel arranged each other. The pedicels envelop most of the glomerular capillaries by interdigitating with those processes from neighboring podocytes. Interdigitation leave the narrow clefts, 20 ~ 40 nm in width, known as filtration slits, between the adjacent pedicels. Filtration slits are covered by a thin filtration slit diaphragm, which extends between neighboring pedicels and acts as a part of the filtration barrier (Fig. 15-6).
- ◆ Parietal layer: The parietal layer of Bowman capsule is a single layer of simple squamous epithelium, which is continuous with the visceral layer at the vascular pole and with the renal tubules at the urinary pole.

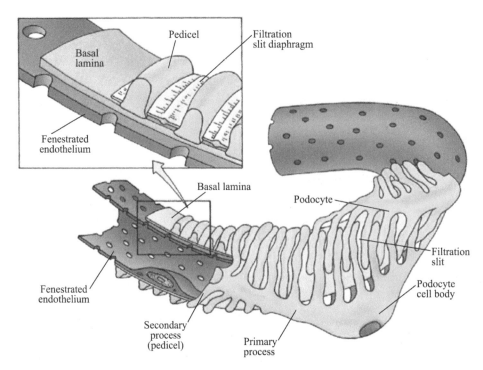

Fig15-6   Diagram of filtration barrier

Filtration barrier is composed of the fenestrated endothelium of the glomerular capillaries, the fused basal lamina between the endothelial cells the parietal layer of Bowman capsule, and the slit diaphragms between the pedicles. The barrier permits the passage of the small molecules, such as water, ions, glucose, amino acids, small-sized proteins and urea from the bloodstream into the Bowman space.

Filtration at the glomerulus selects molecules based on ionic charges and sizes. Among similarly sized molecules, those with a net positive charge are filtered more readily than those with a net neutral or negative charge. The filtrate leaving the Bowman capsule is very similar to blood plasma except the large-molecule proteins as it passes into the proximal convoluted tubule.

Because the basal lamina traps larger macromolecules, it would become clogged were it not continuously phagocytosed by intraglomerular mesangial cells and replenished by both the podocytes and glomerular endothelial cells.

ii . Renal tubule

The renal tubule is continuous with the urinary pole of a Bowman capsule. The tubule is divided into three segments: the proximal tubule, the thin limb of Henle loop, and the distal tubule. The filtrate from the glomerulus enters the proximal tubule, and this takes a coiled course in the cortex before straightening. The coiled portion and the straight portion are the proximal convoluted tubule and the pars recta of the proximal tubule, respectively. The pars recta of the proximal tubule, the thin limb and the pars recta of the distal tubule constitute the

U-shaped loop, Henle loop. The Henle loop initiates from proximal convoluted tubule in the cortex towards the medulla, then returns to the cortex and continues as a distal convoluted tubule which eventually drains into a collecting tubule. (Fig. 15-2, Fig. 15-4 and Fig. 15-7)

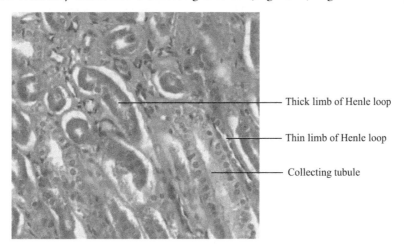

Thick limb of Henle loop

Thin limb of Henle loop

Collecting tubule

Fig. 15-7   Section of the kidney showing the medulla

A. Proximal tubule   The proximal tubule has two regions: the proximal convoluted tubule and the pars recta (descending thick limb of Henle loop).

The proximal tubules are lined by simple cuboidal epithelial cells. These cells have an elaborate striated border on the luminal surface, an intricate system of interlocking and interwoven lateral cell processes, and extensive basal plasma membrane infoldings. The lateral cell membranes are usually indistinguishable with the light microscope.

About 80% of NaCl and water from the glomerular filtrate is reabsorbed by the epithelium of the proximal tubules and transported into the connective tissue stroma by cells of the proximal tubule. By the aid of sodium potassium adenosine triphosphatase ($Na^+-K^+ATPase$) in the cell membranes, Na^+ and Cl^- reabsorbed from the filtrate and potassium (K^+) is excreted into the lumen. Water absorption is followed by to maintain osmotic equilibrium, mostly through tight junctions between the cuboidal cells as well as through aquaporin 1 channels located in the basolateral cell membrane. In addition, all of the glucose, amino acids, and protein in the filtrate are reabsorbed by the proximal tubule. Moreover, the proximal tubule excretes H^+ into the urine and also eliminates the organic solutes (e.g. catecholamines, bile salts, and oxalate), drugs (e.g. penicillin), and toxins from the body.

B. Thin limb of henle loop   The thin limb of Henle loop is lined by simple squamous epithelial cells. The length of the thin segments varies with the location of the nephron. In cortical nephrons, the thin segment is short and may be completely absent. Juxtamedullary nephrons have much longer thin segments and they form a hairpin-like loop that extends deep into the medulla.

The nuclei of the cells bulge into the lumen of the tubule; hence, in paraffin section, these limbs resemble capillaries in cross-section. They may be distinguished from capillaries, in that their epithelial lining cells are slightly thicker, their nuclei stain less densely, and their lumens contain no blood cells.

The thin limb is highly permeable to water due to the presence of numerous aquaporin 1 water channels; it is moderately permeable to urea, and slightly permeable to sodium, chloride, and other ions.

C. Distal tubule   The distal tubule is subdivided into the pars recta (ascending thick limb of Henle loop) and the distal convoluted tubule.

The pars recta of the distal tubule joins the thin limb of Henle loop and ascends straight up through the medulla to reach the cortex. The low cuboidal epithelial cells have centrally placed oval nuclei and a few short microvilli. The lateral sides of the cells interdigitate with each other. Basal plasma membrane infoldings are much more extensive, whereas the number of mitochondria is greater in these cells than in those of the proximal convoluted tubules. Moreover, these cells form abundant zonulae occludentes with their neighboring cells.

Distal convoluted tubules are shorter than proximal convoluted tubules in length. In paraffin sections, the lumens of these tubules are wide open, the cytoplasm of the low cuboidal lining epithelium is paler than those of proximal convoluted tubules, and because the cells are narrower, more nuclei are apparent in tubular cross-section. The ultrastructure of these cells demonstrates a clear, pale cytoplasm with a few blunt apical microvilli. Nuclei are round and apically located, having one or two dense nucleoli. Mitochondria are not as numerous, and the basal plasma membrane infoldings are not as extensive as those of the proximal convoluted tubule.

The distal convoluted tubule is impermeable to water and urea. However, in the basolateral cell membrane presents highly active Na^+-K^+ ATPase, which in response to the hormone aldosterone, can actively reabsorb almost all of the remaining Na^+ (and, passively, Cl^-) from the lumen of the tubule into the renal interstitium; and expel the K^+ and the H^+ into the lumen, thus controlling the body's extracellular fluid potassium level and the acidity of urine, respectively.

II. Collecting duct

Collecting ducts are not part of the nephron. They have different embryological origins, and it is only later in development that they meet the nephron and join it to form a continuous structure. The distal convoluted ducts of several nephrons join to form a short connecting tubule that leads into the collecting duct. Collecting ducts have three regions: cortical, medullary and papillary collecting tubule

The collecting duct is composed of the simple cuboidal epithelium. The epithelial cells have oval, centrally located nuclei; a few small mitochondria; and short sparse microvilli. The basal membranes of these cells display numerous infoldings. The cell membranes are clearly evident with the light microscope. These cells possess numerous aquaporin-2 channels that are very sensitive to antidiuretic hormone (ADH) and become completely permeable to water, thereby permitting themselves to reabsorb water from the filtrate, thus concentrating urine.

The typical epithelial cells of the segments of the urinary duct are shown in Fig. 15-8.

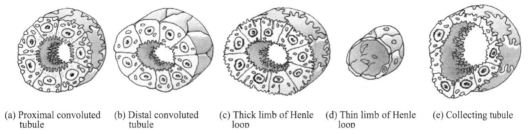

(a) Proximal convoluted   (b) Distal convoluted   (c) Thick limb of Henle   (d) Thin limb of Henle   (e) Collecting tubule
    tubule   tubule   loop   loop

Fig. 15-8   Diagram of epithelial cells of renal tubules and collecting tubule

III. Juxtaglomerular apparatus

The juxtaglomerular apparatus is an important structure that regulates the balance of ions and the volume of the body fluid, consisting of the macula densa of the distal tubule, juxtaglomerular cells of the adjacent afferent glomerular arteriole, and the extraglomerular mesangial cells (Fig. 15-9).

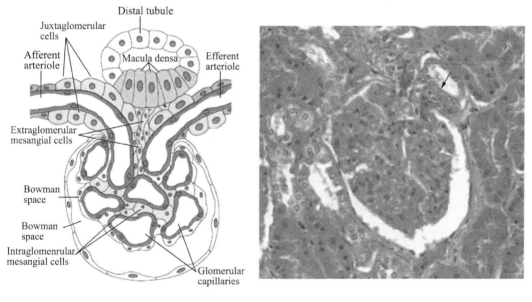

(a) Diagram of juxtaglomerular apparatus   (b) Section of the kidney showing the macula densa(arrow)

Fig. 15-9   Juxtaglomerular apparatus

i . Macula densa

The macula densa is the specialized epithelial cells of distal convoluted tubules. The cells are tall, narrow, pale cells with centrally placed nuclei. Because of the narrowness of these cells, the densely staining nuclei are near to each other so that they appear as a dense spot. These cells sense the concentration of ions and the flowing volume of the filtrate passing by.

ii . Juxtaglomerular cells

The juxtaglomerular cells, modified smooth muscle cells located in the tunica media of afferent glomerular arterioles. The nuclei of these cells are round instead of elongated. Juxtaglomerular cells contain granules of renin. Via its effects on the liver and lungs, renin controls the production of angiotensin which in turn stimulates the production of aldosterone by the adrenal glands and causes the contraction of small arteries; and as the results, the reabsorbing Na^+ and expelling K^+ are promoted, and the blood pressure is elevated.

iii. Extraglomerular mesangial cells

The extraglomerular mesangial cells occupy the space bounded by the afferent arteriole, macula densa, efferent arteriole, and vascular pole of the renal corpuscle. These cells are probably contiguous with the intraglomerular mesangial cells and they function as the messenger transfer between the macula densa and the juxtaglomerular cells.

Ⅳ. Renal interstitium

The renal interstitium is a flimsy scant amount of loose connective tissue housing three types of cells: fibroblasts, macrophages, and interstitial cells. Interstitial cells appear to be situated like the rungs of a ladder, one on top of the other. The cells synthesize medullipin Ⅰ, a substance that is converted in the liver to medullipin Ⅱ, a potent vasodilator that lowers blood pressure; and they also produce erythropoietin (EPO), which acts on bone marrow stem cells to promote differentiation into red blood cells.

Ⅴ. Blood circulation in kidney

The two kidneys receive an extremely extensive blood supply via the large renal arteries, direct branches of the abdominal aorta. Before entering the hilum of the kidney, the renal artery bifurcates into an anterior and a posterior division, which, in turn, subdivide to form the segmental arteries (Fig. 15-10).

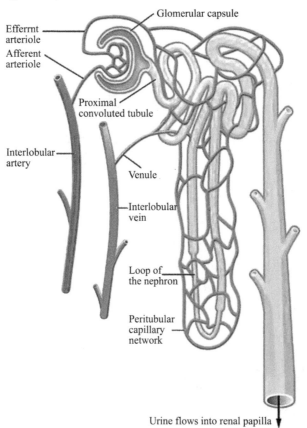

Fig. 15-10   Diagram of blood circulation of kidney

The first subdivisions of the segmental arteries are lobar arteries, one for each lobe of the kidney. These in turn branch to form two or three interlobar arteries, which travel between the renal pyramids to the corticomedullary junction. Hereby, these arteries are arcuate arteries. The terminal branches of the arcuate arteries ascend into the cortex, forming interlobular arteries. The afferent glomerular arterioles are arised from the interlobular arteries.

Efferent glomerular arterioles from cortical nephrons are short and branch to form a system of capillaries, the peritubular capillary network. This capillary bed supplies the entire cortical labyrinth. Each efferent glomerular arteriole gives rise to hairpin-like the vasa recta, closely follows and wraps around the Henle loop and the collecting tubule, is essential in the physiology of urine concentration. Thus, the kidney possesses a dual capillary bed, one responsible for the formation of the filtrate, the glomerulus with a high hydrostatic pressure and the second, the peritubular capillary bed with a low hydrostatic pressure. This hydrostatic pressure differential permits the exceptionally efficient reabsorption of the fluid conserved by the renal tubules.

The arcuate veins receive blood from the cortex via the stellate veins and interlobular veins and from the medulla via the venae rectae; arcuate veins are drained by the interlobar veins that deliver their blood into the renal vein.

15.2   Urinary Bladder

The urinary bladder is an organ for storing urine until discharge. The bladder has a mucosa composed of a transitional epithelium, the lamina propria, smooth muscle layer, which is enveloped by a serosa on its posterior aspect, whereas its anterior aspect has an adventitia that causes the bladder to adhere to the anterior abdominal wall (Fig. 15-11).

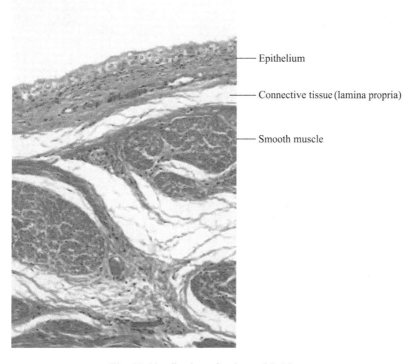

Epithelium

Connective tissue (lamina propria)

Smooth muscle

Fig. 15-11   Section of urinary bladder

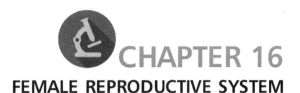

CHAPTER 16
FEMALE REPRODUCTIVE SYSTEM

Female reproductive system consists of paired ovaries and reproductive tract, comprising paired oviducts, a uterus and a vagina. At puberty, hormones from the pituitary gland initiate developmental changes which are prerequisites for reproduction. In contrast to the male reproductive system, the female system after puberty in humans is regulated by hormones secreted by the pituitary gland on a monthly cyclical basis. The cycle of activity begins at puberty and is manifested by the onset of menstruation. The time when menstruation begins is known as the menarche and it occurs between 9 and 15 years of age. During each monthly menstrual cycle, female oocytes differentiate and usually a single, mature oocyte is shed from an ovary, a process described as ovulation. The ability to produce a haploid gamete (an ovum), conceive, support one or more developing fetuses and give birth continues from puberty until the menopause. During the menopause, which may begin between 45 and 50 years of age, the menstrual cycles and ovulation become irregular and then cease.

16.1 Ovaries

The ovaries are the solid, almond-shaped organs, located within the pelvis. Their size and histological appearance differ during menstrual cycles, pregnancy, and postmenopausal period. Ovaries are covered by the germinal epithelium or ovarian surface epithelium. Under the surface epithelium is a dense fibrous connective tissue, the tunica albuginea, which encapsulates the whole ovary. An ovary is divided into an outer cortex and an inner medulla. (Fig. 16-1)

16.1.1 Cortex of the ovary

The cortex has ovarian follicles in various stages of development and stoma. Ovarian follicles comprise an oogonium, or a developing oocyte, surrounded by epithelial cells. Between puberty and the menopause, ovarian follicles vary widely in appearance and size as they are in various stages of development. The stoma house fibroblast-like stromal cells. Some stromal cells are irregularly distributed in whorls in the cortex and others lie around developing follicles as layers known as theca. Some cells in the theca differentiate and are able to secrete steroid hormones.

In childhood, the cortex contains numerous primordial follicles; in sexually mature women, corpora lutea form at sites of ruptured follicles. Ovaries at birth hold about 4 million primary oocytes, which developed from oogonia; by puberty, about 40 thousand oocytes remain after degeneration or atresia. In women, an ovum is liberated from an ovary via ovulation about every 28 days. Moreover ovaries produce the hormones estrogen and progesterone.

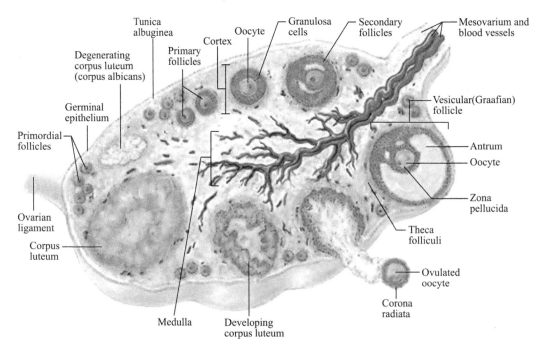

Fig. 16-1　Diagram of an ovary

I . Development of ovarian follicles

Ovarian follicles consist of an oocyte and surrounding epithelial layer of follicular cells. By birth, all oogonia have become primary oocytes, which have reached prophase of the first division of meiosis. Follicles in the cortex may be resting, or primordial; maturing or growing (known as primary and secondary follicles); or mature (Graafian).

i . Primordial follicles

Primordial follicles are just under the tunica albuginea and have not yet begun to develop. They contain a primary oocyte, measuring about 25 μm in diameter, with an eccentric nucleus and a prominent nucleolus. One layer of squamous epithelial cells, the follicular cells, surrounds it. A thin basal lamina lies on the outer surface of these cells and separates them from surrounding connective tissue stroma. (Fig. 16-2)

ii . Growing follicles

After puberty, about 20 primordial follicles become activated monthly during menstrual cycles. Usually, only a few follicles among them become dominant and move to the stage by becoming a growing follicle, first primary follicle, then secondary follicle.

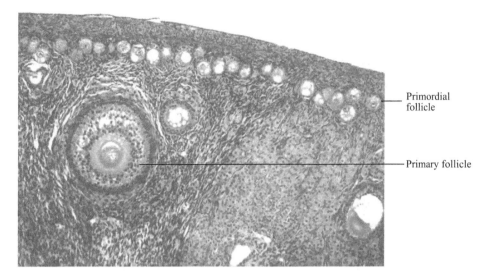

Fig. 16-2   Section of the ovary (middle magnification)

A. Primary follicle   This follicle is slightly larger, with an oocyte, $40 \sim 45$ μm in diameter, containing a large clear nucleus with distinct nucleolus. Surrounding follicular cells undergo cell division and become cuboidal. Their cytoplasm assumes a granular appearance, so the cells are now known as granulosa cells, which are surrounded by a basal lamina. Stromal cells adjacent to the follicle differentiate into a concentric sheath of theca interna cells. At this stage when the granulosa cells are present one-layered, the follicle is described as unilaminar primary follicles.

At this stage, the follicles are described as unilaminar primary follicles.

Unilaminar follicles become multilaminar follicles as mitotic activity is high in granulosa cells and the new cells form layers around each developing primary oocyte. During this time, the primary oocyte enlarges considerably and a prominent deposit of condensed material known as the zona pellucida appears between the oocyte and the granulosa cells (Fig. 16-3).

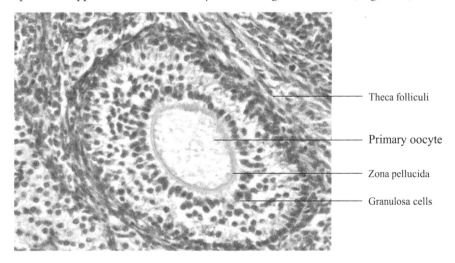

Fig. 16-3   Section of the ovary showing the primary follicle(high magnification)

Stromal cells around each primary follicle form two layers during this phase: the theca interna and theca externa. The inner theca is well vascularised whereas the outer theca is composed of fibrous connective tissue. Luteinising hormone (LH) from the pituitary gland stimulates cells of theca to produce steroids. These steroids are converted by granulosa cells into estrogens (female steroid hormones). Estrogens are involved in stimulating the uterus each month (see below) and in the development and maintenance of the secondary sexual characteristics and of the mammary glands.

B. Secondary follicles   Some multilaminar primary follicles develop and enlarge further, under the influence of follicle-stimulating hormone (FSH). The granulosa cells produce fluid, liquor folliculi, which appears in spaces between the granulosa cells. These follicles are described as secondary (antral) follicles (Fig. 16-4). Gradually, the fluid-filled spaces coalesce into a single large space, the antrum, and development proceeds with the formation of a Graafian (mature) follicle.

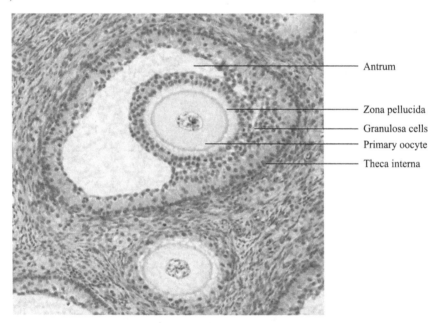

Fig. 16-4   Section of the ovary(middle magnification) showing the secondary follicle

C. Graafian (mature) follicles   As the single antrum enlarges the granulose cells appear as layers around the fluid and the layers become thinner as the follicle enlarges further. The oocyte, surrounded by granulosa cells, bulges into the fluid in the antrum and the whole bulge is known as the cumulus oophorus, which projects into the antrum. One or more layers of granulosa cells are attached to the oocyte as the corona radiata.

Graafian follicles may become very large (2.5 cm in diameter) and bulge from the surface of the ovary prior to ovulation. The primary oocyte, which was arrested in prophase of the first meiotic division, completes the first meiotic division just prior to ovulation. The result is one large secondary oocyte with half the original number of chromosomes (23 in humans) and a small cell, known as the first polar body (also with 23 chromosomes), which degenerates. (Fig. 16-5)

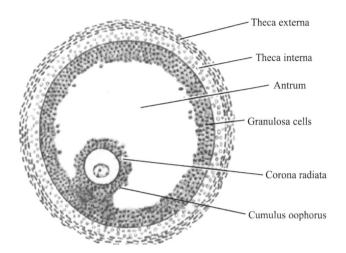

Fig. 16-5   Diagram of Graafian follicle

II. Ovulation

Ovulation usually happens once at the mid-point (~ day 14) of every menstrual cycle. It is the process of rupture of a Graafian follicle whereby a secondary oocyte and the surrounding corona radiata are expelled and away from the surface of the ovary. Ovulation is brought about as the increasing volume of the granulosa cells puts pressure onto the tunica albuginea and surface epithelium of the ovary and also compresses blood vessels in the region. This is coincidental with a breakdown of the wall of the follicle in the same region. The oocyte, granulosa cells forming the corona radiata and fluid burst from the antrum of the follicle and enter the peritoneal cavity and are carried by the opening of the oviduct.

III. Corpus luteum

After ovulation, under the influence of luteinizing hormone, a corpus luteum develops. It forms from the remnants of granulosa cells from the ruptured Graafian follicle, and cells and blood vessels which grow into these remnants from the theca interna. The theca and granulosa cells forming the corpus luteum begin to secrete female steroid hormones, mainly progesterone, as well as estrogens. (Fig. 16-6)

The progesterone secreted by the corpus luteum is essential in preparing the uterus for the possible arrival of a fertilized ovum and the establishment of pregnancy. If pregnancy is established the corpus luteum doubles in size and is an essential source of progesterone during the first months of pregnancy. If fertilization and implantation do not occur, the corpus luteum degenerates, a scar forms from fibroblasts and collagen fibres, and the resultant structure, known as a corpus albicans, persists in the ovary for some time.

IV. Atresia of follicles

Most developing follicles fail to become mature Graafian follicles. Atresia may occur at any stage of follicle development and it involves the death of granulosa cells and the oocyte. Atretic follicles are gradually replaced by scar tissue containing fibroblasts and collagen.

16.1.2 Medulla of the ovary

The medulla is the central core of the ovary and it is surrounded by the cortex except where vessels and nerves are connected to the ovary. The poorly-defined medulla consists of loose connective tissue with many convoluted blood vessels, nerves, and lymphatics. Stromal cells, similar to those in the cortex, are present in the medulla but follicles are not present.

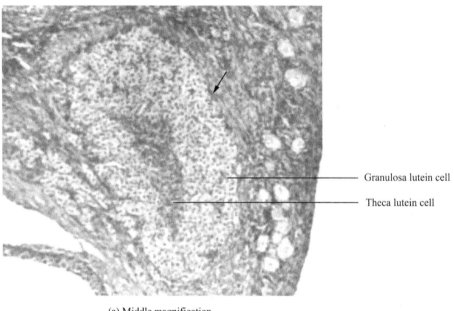

(a) Middle magnification

— Granulosa lutein cell

— Theca lutein cell

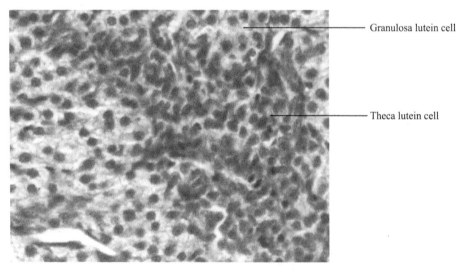

(b) High magnification

Fig. 16-6　Section of the ovary showing the corpus luteum(arrow)

— Granulosa lutein cell

— Theca lutein cell

16.2　Oviduct

Each oviduct in humans is about 10 cm long. The lumen at one end of each tube is open to the peritoneal cavity. This end is formed by frilly, fingerlike projections (fimbriae) of the tube. Fimbriae are important in helping guide the oocyte (released at ovulation into the peritoneal cavity) into the lumen of the oviduct. The other end of the oviduct opens into the uterus. The structure of each oviduct consists of three layers: mucosa, muscularis and serosa.

The inner layer is a mucosa. The mucosa is highly folded and consists of simple columnar epithelial cells on a basement membrane and a thin, supporting connective tissue lamina propria). Some epithelial cells have cilia and others do not. The non-ciliated cells are secretory and the fluid they produce provides an environment in the lumen of the duct in which the (secondary) oocyte and spermatozoa can survive and fertilization can occur. The ciliated cells beat and assist in wafting the oocyte toward the uterus. The fluid in the oviduct and its direction of flow towards the uterus also help to prevent the invasion of microorganisms into the oviduct and the peritoneal cavity. (Fig. 16-7)

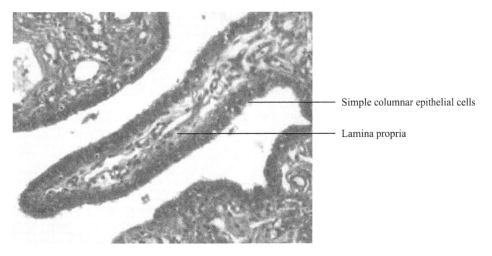

Simple columnar epithelial cells

Lamina propria

Fig. 16-7   Section of the oviduct showing the projection of the mucosa

The middle layer is a muscularis. There are an inner circular and an outer longitudinal layer. Peristaltic contractions of the smooth muscle cells assist in moving the contents of the lumen.

The outer layer is a thin covering of serosa.

16.3   Uterus

In the pelvis, between the urinary bladder and rectum, lies the uterus, a hollow pear-shaped organ with a thick muscular wall and a lumen lined by a mucous membrane. The expanded, upper part of the organ is the body, or corpus. Oviducts enter the wall at the most superior, dome-shaped region, called the fundus. At the narrowest and most inferior part of the organ, the cervix opens into the vagina. The body and fundus are almost identical histologically, but the cervix shows some important structural differences. The wall of the uterus in the body and fundus regions is composed of three layers: endometrium, myometrium and perimetrium. (Fig. 16-8)

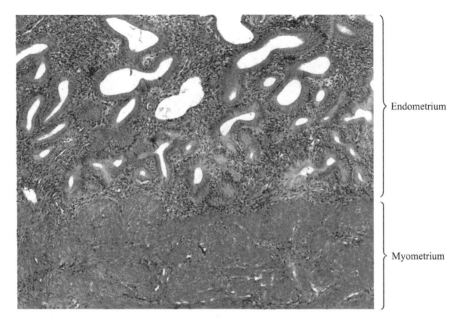

Fig. 16-8   Section of the uterus (low magnification)

16.3.1 Endometrium

This is a mucosa; it forms the inner layer and varies in structure under the influence of estrogens and progesterone. The endometrium has a basal layer and a superficial (functional) layer. A simple, columnar epithelium lines the uterine lumen and branched tubular glands dip deep into the connective tissue of the lamina propria. Some of the epithelial cells are secretory and others have cilia.

Within the superficial layer there are helical arteries. These supply the endometrium as it increases in thickness in response to the hormonal changes occurring during the menstrual cycle. (Fig. 16-9)

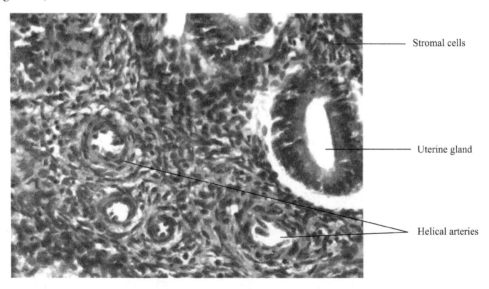

Fig. 16-9   Section of the uterus(high magnification) showing the endometrium

The basal layer of the endometrium is a relatively narrow region, though highly significant, since it is this layer that undergoes cellular proliferation and replaces the superficial layer shed at menstruation.

16.3.2 Myometrium

Myometrium is composed of three layers of smooth muscle. Longitudinal muscle makes up the inner and outer layers, whereas the richly vascularized middle layer contains mostly circularly arranged smooth muscle bundles. As the uterus narrows toward the cervix, the smooth muscle tissue diminishes and is replaced by fibrous connective tissue. At the cervix, the myometrium is composed of dense irregular collagenous connective tissue.

16.3.3 Perimetrium

Because the uterus is tipped anteriorly and lies against the bladder, much of its anterior portion is covered by adventitia (connective tissue without an epithelial covering), thus, this area is retroperitoneal. The fundus and posterior portion of the body are covered by a serosa, composed of a layer of squamous mesothelial cells resting on areolar connective tissue; therefore, this area is intraperitoneal.

16.4 Menstrual Cycle

The menstrual cycle is a sequence of morphologic and functional changes during the reproductive ages of female that occurs every 28 days in the absence of pregnancy. The endometrium and ovaries undergo cyclic changes resulting from interplay of hormones produced by the pituitary, ovarian follicles, and corpus luteum. Phases in the cycle are below:

16.4.1 Menstrual phase (days 1 ~4)

Menstruation, which begins on the day that bleeding from the uterus starts, occurs if fertilization does not take place. In this case, the corpus luteum becomes nonfunctional about 14 days after ovulation, thus reducing the levels of progesterone and estrogen. A couple of days before bleeding begins, the functionalis layer of the endometrium becomes deprived of blood as the coiled helical arteries are intermittently constricted. After 2 days or so, the helical arteries become permanently constricted, reducing oxygen to the functional layer, leading to a shutdown of the glands, invasion by leukocytes, ischemia, and eventual necrosis of the functional layer. Shortly thereafter, the helical arteries dilate again; however, because these helical arteries have been weakened by the previous events, they rupture. The disgorged blood removes patches of the functional layer to be discharged.

The basal layer is preserved to restore the endometrium during the follicular phase. At this stage, production of estrogen is low but that of FSH is maximal, leading to follicular growth in ovaries.

16.4.2 Follicular or proliferative phase (days 4 ~ 15)

It begins just after menstruation and ends after ovulation. Rapid regeneration of the endometrium begins from the narrow zone left after menstruation. The epithelium in the basal portions of the uterine glands replicates and grows to cover the raw mucosal surface. Numerous mitoses are seen in columnar epithelial cells of the glands, and connective tissue cells in the stroma multiply and rebuild the lamina propria. Uterine glands lengthen and become closely packed. They are simple and straight and lead directly from the base to the mucosal surface. Spiral arteries also grow from the stratum basale into more superficial regenerated tissue. The proliferative and repair activities are regulated indirectly by follicle-stimulating hormone (FSH). (Fig. 16-10a)

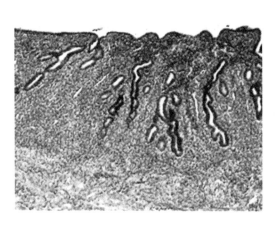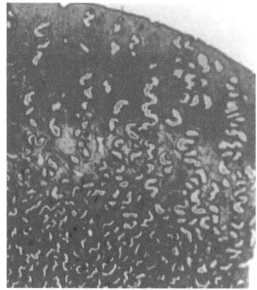

(a) Showing the endometrium in the proliferative phage (b) Showing the endometrium in the secretory phage

Fig. 16-10   Section of the uterus(low magnification)

16.4.3   Luteal or secretory phase (days 15 ~ 28)

This phase begins after ovulation (on day 14) and lasts until menstruation (i. e. from day 15 to day 28). After ovulation, luteinising hormone (LH) stimulates the formation of the corpus luteum, which secretes progesterone. Under the influence of progesterone, the whole endometrium becomes thicker and oedematous; meanwhile the glands deepen and become saw-toothed in shape. The epithelial cells accumulate glycogen and secrete glycoproteins into the lumen, activities which could provide nourishment for a developing blastocyst. The timing of these events is also essential in preparing the endometrium for the blastocyst, particularly as the uterine secretions will nourish the developing embryo prior to the formation of the placenta. (Fig. 16-10b)

16.4.4   Hormonal control of the menstrual cycle

The hypothalamus secretes gonadotropin-releasing hormone (GnRH). In response to GnRH, the adenohypophysis secrets FSH and LH. In response to FSH, the development of a secondary follicle to a Graafian follicle is stimulated in the ovary. The granulosa cells within the secondary follicle and Graafian follicle secrete estrogen (E). In response to estrogen, endometrium of the uterus enters the proliferative phase. In response to LH surge in the middle of the cycle (around day 14), ovulation occurs. After ovulation, the granulose lutein cells of the corpus luteum secrete progesterone (P). Progesterone impacts upon the endometrium and results in its entering the secretory phase. The high levels of E and P inhibit the secretion of FSH and LH by hypophysis, and the down-regulated level of FSH and LH degenerate the corpus luteum. If not pregnant, the corpus luteum maintains for about 12 ~ 14 days. Due to the degeneration of corpus luteum, the endometrium undergoes ischemia, necrosis and shedding-off. Meanwhile, the down-regulated E and P from the corpus luteum reduce the inhibition of secretion of FSH and LH. Thus the recovered level of FSH and LH stimulate a new batch of ovarian follicles to develop and another menstrual cycle starts.

The relationship between the ovaries and the uterus is shown in Fig. 16-11.

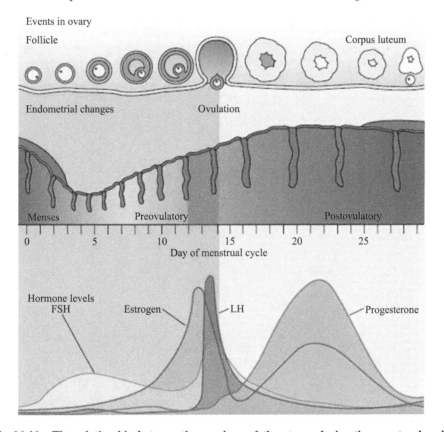

Fig. 16-11   The relationship between the ovaries and the uterus during the menstrual cycle

CHAPTER 17
MALE REPRODUCTIVE SYSTEM

The male reproductive system consists of the two testes suspended in the scrotum, a system of genital ducts, associated glands, and external genitals.

The testes are responsible for the formation of the male gametes, known as spermatozoa, as well as for the synthesis of the male sex hormone.

After spermatozoa are produced in the testes, they travel a long, tortuous route: from seminiferous tubules to the rete testis, efferent ductules (ductuli efferentes), epididymis, vas deferens, ejaculatory ducts, and to the single urethra and penis. Accessory glands include seminal vesicles, prostate and bulbourethral glands. Their secretions, together with the sperm, form semen and are essential to sperm function and survival.

Three key functions of this system are production of spermatozoa, delivery of these cells via semen into the female reproductive tract, and production of testosterone.

17.1　Testes

The testes reside outside the body cavity in the scrotum. Testes are invested by distinct three layers, from outer to inner respectively are: tunica vaginalis, tunica albuginea (thick dense connective tissue), and tunica vasculosa. The tunica vaginalis is serous membrane that covers the testes. The tunica albuginea consists of thick dense connective tissue, and so called because it appears white in life. The tunica vasculosa consists of a plexus of blood vessels, held together by connective tissue.

The thickening tunica albuginea along the posterior aspect of the testes form mediastinum, which projects incomplete septa radially to divide the testis into lobules.

Each lobule contains several convoluted seminiferous tubules, whose germinal epithelium produces male germ cells known as spermatozoa. The stroma between the seminiferous tubules are interstitial tissue, housing interstitial cells, also known as Leydig cells, which produce testosterone, the hormone responsible for male secondary sex characteristics and required for the generation of spermatozoa. (Fig. 17-1)

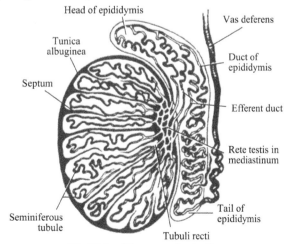

Fig. 17-1　Diagram of a testis

17.1.1 Seminiferous tubules

Seminiferous tubules are highly convoluted tubules. The wall of the seminiferous tubule is composed of a thin connective tissue layer, the tunica propria, and a thick seminiferous epithelium. The seminiferous epithelium (or germinal epithelium) is several cell layers thick and is composed of two types of cells: spermatogenic cells in various stages of maturation and Sertoli cells. (Fig. 17-2)

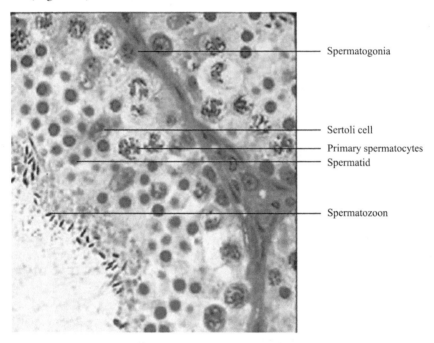

Fig. 17-2　Section of the testis showing the seminiferous tubules

I . Spermatogenic cells and spermatogenesis

The spermatogenesis is the process by which spermatogonia divide and differentiate into spermatozoa. Spermatogenic cells include five successive cells. (Fig. 17-3)

i . Spermatogonia

They are located adjacent to the basal membrane. Spermatogonia are small cells with the normal number of chromosomes (46, comprising 22 homologous pairs and two sex chromosomes). Some of the new cells formed by mitosis remain in the basal layer as spermatogonia (Type A), and other spermatogonia (Type B) divide mitotically to give rise to primary spermatocytes and enter meiosis.

ii . Primary spermatocytes

They replicate the DNA in their chromosomes prior to cell division and get enlarged, containing diploid (2n) chromosomes (44 +XY) and tetraploid (4n) DNA. Then undergo the first meiotic division. Each pair of homologous chromosomes are separated and given to the two daughter cells. The result of this division is the production of two secondary spermatocytes each with only half the original number of chromosomes (i. e. 23).

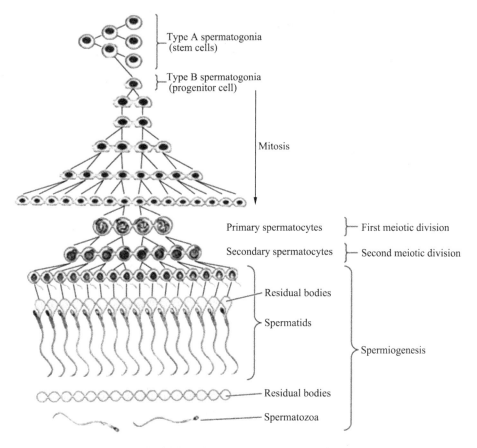

Fig. 17-3 Diagram of spermatogenesis

iii. Secondary spermatocytes

They are smaller cells near the lumen, with round nucleus, and few in number. They contain haploid (1n) chromosomes (22 +X or Y) and 2n DNA, and immediately undergo the second meiosis (chromatids separate) producing the spermatids. The second meiotic division occurs rapidly. The chromosomes then split and separate into two new cells, known as spermatids. As this cell division is rapid, few cells in any one histological section are in this phase. Each resulting spermatid has 23 chromosomes with the haploid amount of DNA. This is half the number of chromosomes and half the DNA in spermatogonia. Separation of cytoplasm during meiosis is incomplete and spermatids derived from one spermatogonium are partially joined together. This is thought to aid synchrony of their progression through the next stage.

iv. Spermatids and spermiogenesis

Spermatids are the smallest, round or ellipsoid cells close to the lumen, haploid (1n) in the number of chromosomes and in the amount of DNA. During this stage of spermiogenesis, spermatids differentiate and each forms one spermatozoon. The spherical spermatids change in form and shed cytoplasm as they become highly differentiated spermatozoa. They do not divide, and transform from round cells into tadpole-like spermatozoa by spermiogenesis. Spermiogenesis includes following changes:

◆ The nucleus becomes condensed and elongated.

- Golgi apparatus transforms into acrosomal vesicle and then acrosome.
- One of centrioles migrates to a position opposite developing acrosome and forms the flagellum (axoneme).
- Mitochondria move and aggregate around proximal part of the flagellum forming a sheath.
- Much of cytoplasm is no longer required and cast off as residual bodies.

v. Spermatozoa

A mature spermatozoon has a head and a tail. The head is pear-shaped, flattened and contains condensed nucleus (22 + X or Y). The anterior 2/3 portion of the head is covered by the cap-like acrosome, which contains hydrolytic enzymes in it and is important for fertilization. (Fig. 17-4)

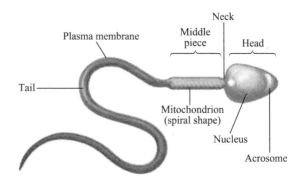

Fig. 17-4   Diagram of a spermatozoon

The tail is long and slender, and has the "9 +2" arrangement of microtubules characteristic of cilia, and these provide the motive force which allows spermatozoa to swim. It is subdivided into four segments:

- The neck is very short and contains one centriole.
- The middle has a sheath of mitochondria which provides the energy for motility.
- The principal has a fibrous sheath providing support and protection.
- The terminal (end-piece) contains only the axoneme.

As spermatozoa develop, the head regions remain in the epithelium but the tail regions extend into the lumen of the seminiferous tubule. Eventually, spermatozoa pass into the lumen and fluid secreted by Sertoli cells aids their transport.

The spermatozoa in the testes appear morphologically mature but functionally immature, that is, they are non-motile and do not fertilize the ovum.

II. Sertoli cells

Sertoli cells play a critical role in support and maturation of spermatozoa. These columnar cells, with borders that are hard to distinguish, extend from the basement membrane to the lumen of the seminiferous tubule. Their apices bear crypt-like recesses that hold spermatids until release of newly formed spermatozoa into the lumen. Each cell has a jagged, euchromatic nucleus with a prominent nucleolus. Adjacent cells are linked by basolateral tight junctions, such that the epithelium is divided into basal and abluminal compartments. The resulting blood-testis permeability barrier separates spermatogonia and primary spermatocytes from more apical secondary spermatocytes and spermatids. Contents in the seminiferous tubule lumen are thus isolated from circulating antigens, thereby protecting spermatocytes and spermatids from autoimmune reactions and blood-borne substances. (Fig. 17-5)

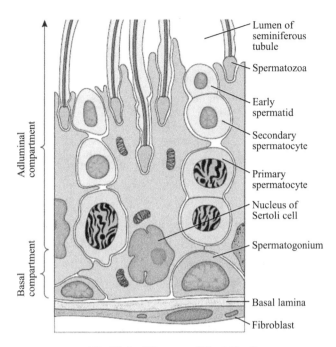

Fig. 17-5   Diagram of Sertoli cells

Sertoli cells phagocytose spermatid remnants and secrete fluid and many substances, including androgen-binding protein (ABP), essential for spermatozoa survival. Tight junctions between Sertoli cells separate basal compartments and abluminal compartments. The basal compartments are close to basal lamina and house the spermatogonia; the abluminal compartments are close to the lumen and house the developing spermatogenic cells. Cell junctions may adjust to the changes in junctional architecture as spermatozoa move toward the lumen. The extensive cytoskeletal network of Sertoli cells helps provide for spermatozoa movement.

17.1.2 Interstitial tissue and Leydig cells

Interstitial connective tissue consists of vascularized connective tissue with clusters of hormone-producing Leydig cells. Leydig cells are endocrine cells in the loose connective tissue around seminiferous tubules and they secrete mainly testosterone (Fig. 17-6). The Leydig cells are stimulated to produce and secrete testosterone by LH secreted by cells in the anterior pituitary gland. Testosterone

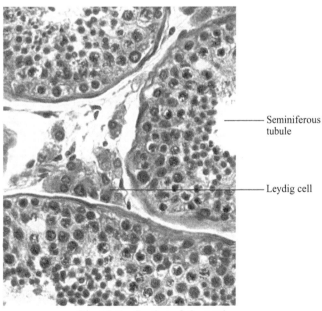

Fig. 17-6   Section of the testis

enters the circulation and stimulates secondary sexual characteristics including skeletal muscle development and the pattern of hair growth. However, circulating levels of testosterone are insufficient to maintain spermatogenesis. Testosterone levels in the testis are kept high enough to stimulate spermatogenesis as the androgen-binding protein (ABP) secreted by Sertoli cells binds testosterone in the testis. Another hormone from anterior pituitary cells, FSH, stimulates Sertoli cells to secrete ABP.

17.1.3 Tubuli recti and rete testis

The both ends of seminiferous tubules are the straight regions (tubuli recti) through which fluid and spermatozoa leave. The tubuli recti drain into a meshwork of spaces, lined by cuboidal epithelium, known as the rete testis. The rete is embedded in the connective tissue, mediastinum, which extends to the tunica albuginea. In the mediastinum, seminiferous tubules empty into tubuli recti and rete testis, which coalesce to form efferent ductules. These ducts drain testicular fluid and spermatozoa to the proximal part of the epididymis. The rete testis is a labyrinthine network of collecting chambers of simple cuboidal epithelium. (Fig. 17-7)

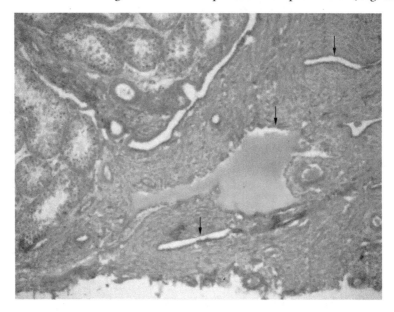

Fig. 17-7   Section of the testis showing the rete testis(arrows)

17.1.4 The hormonal control of the male reproductive system

The hypothalamus secret gonadotropin-releasing hormone (GnRH) and it stimulates the adenohypophysis secreting follicle-stimulating hormone (FSH) and luteinizing hormone (LH). FSH binds to the receptors on the Sertoli cells, which stimulates the synthesis of androgen-binding protein (ABP). The Sertoli cells secrete inhibin, which inhibits FSH secretion. LH binds to LH receptors on the Leydig cells, which stimulates the secretion of testosterone. Testosterone circulates in the blood stimulate and maintain the secondary sexual characteristics and also bind ABP to maintain the high level of testosterone necessary for the spermatogenesis. The testosterone in the blood give rise a negative feedback to the GnRH produced by hypothalamus, thus the levels of testosterone is balanced (Fig. 17-8).

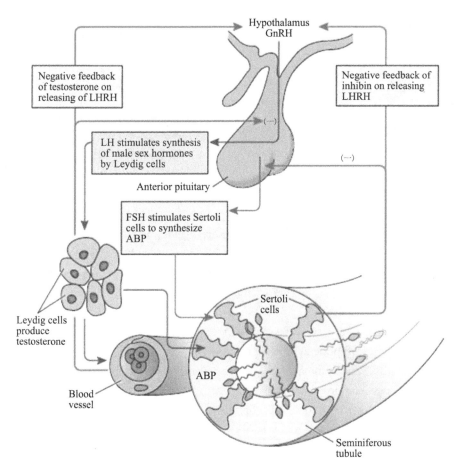

Fig. 17-8 The hormonal control of the male reproductive system

17.2 Epididymis

The epididymis caps the posterior part of each testis, its main component being a tightly packed, tortuous duct. The epididymis is divided into three parts: an initial (head) segment, a body (the main part of the duct), and a caudal (tail) region. The head consists of tightly coiled parts of efferent ductules. Several cross and oblique views of the same duct are usually seen in histologic sections-evidence of the extremely convoluted nature of the duct. The head receives efferent ductules that emerge from the rete testis and is engaged primarily in absorption of fluid and particulate matter. The efferent ductules are lined by ciliated columnar epithelium; the cilia beat in the direction of the epididymis and may aid movement of spermatozoa. Duct of epididymis is a single, narrow, tightly-coiled tube connecting the efferent ductules from the rear of each testicle to its vas deferens. Through the epididymis, which is a long storage duct, spermatozoa pass slowly, their journey taking one to several weeks. In transit, spermatozoa mature and acquire motility and fertilizing capacity. (Fig. 17-1, Fig. 17-9)

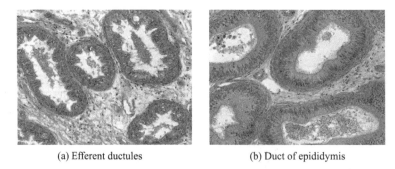

| (a) Efferent ductules | (b) Duct of epididymis |

Fig. 17-9　Section of the epididymis

17.3　Prostate Gland

The prostate gland, the largest of the accessory glands, is pierced by the urethra and the ejaculatory ducts. The slender capsule of the gland is composed of richly vascularized, dense irregular collagenous cells. The connective tissue stroma of the gland is derived from the capsule and is, therefore, also enriched by smooth muscle fibers. This gland is arranged in three layers: mucosal, submucosal and main.

Each tubuloacinar gland has its own duct that delivers the secretory product into the prostatic urethra. The components of the prostate gland are lined by a simple to pseudostratified columnar epithelium. The lumina of the tubuloacinar glands frequently house round to oval prostatic concretions, composed of calcified glycoproteins (Fig. 17-10). The significance of these concretions is not understood. The prostatic secretion is a serous, white fluid rich in lipids, proteolytic enzymes, acid phosphatase, fibrinolysin, and citric acid. The formation, synthesis, and release of the prostatic secretions are regulated by testosterone.

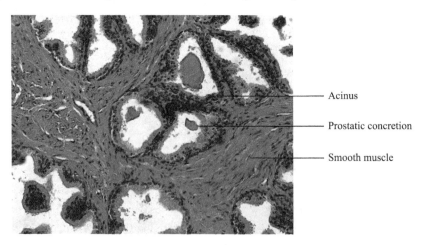

    ——— Acinus

    ——— Prostatic concretion

    ——— Smooth muscle

Fig. 17-10　Section of the prostate gland

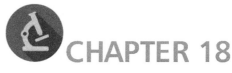

CHAPTER 18
EYE AND EAR

18.1 Eye

The eyes are located within the hollow bony orbits of the skull. The wall of eyeball has three concentric coats. The mainly protective outer fibrous layer (tunica fibrosa) consists of an opaque sclera posteriorly and a transparent cornea anteriorly. The middle vascular coat, or uvea (tunica vasculosa), comprises choroid, ciliary body, and iris. The inner layer, the retina, consists of a small anteriorly nonneural region. At the posterior, it becomes the neural retina. The multilayer neural retina contains specialized photoreceptors and other retinal cells. Optic nerve fibers from the retina exit posteriorly at the optic disc (blind spot). The interior ocular chambers are the small anterior and posterior chambers, containing transparent fluid, the aqueous humor and the vitreous body. (Fig. 18-1)

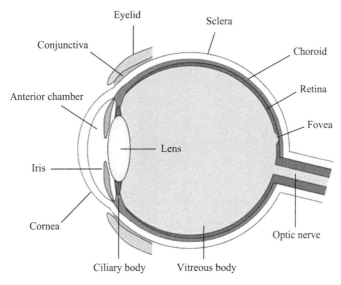

Fig. 18-1 Diagram of eyeball

18.1.1 Wall of eyeball

I. Tunica fibrosa

The tunica fibrosa is composed of the sclera and the cornea. The external fibrous tunic of the eye, the tunica fibrosa, is divided into the sclera and the cornea. The white, opaque sclera covers the posterior five sixths of the eyeball, whereas the colorless, transparent cornea covers the anterior one sixth of the eyeball.

i . Cornea

The cornea is the transparent, avascular, and highly innervated anterior portion of the fibrous tunic that bulges out anteriorly from the eyeball. The cornea is composed of the histologically distinct five layers: corneal epithelium, Bowman membrane, stroma, Descemet membrane and corneal endothelium. (Fig. 18-2)

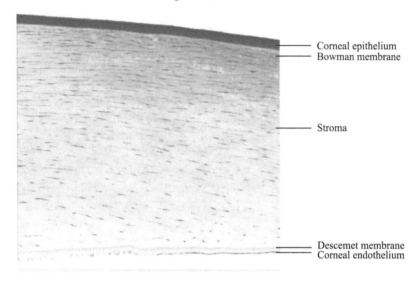

Corneal epithelium
Bowman membrane

Stroma

Descemet membrane
Corneal endothelium

Fig. 18-2   Section of the cornea

◆ Corneal epithelium: The corneal epithelium, the continuation of the conjunctiva (a mucous membrane covering the anterior sclera and lining the internal surface of the eyelids), is a stratified, squamous, nonkeratinized epithelium, composed of five to seven layers of cells. Damage to the cornea is repaired rapidly as cells migrate to the defect to cover the injured region. Subsequently, mitotic activity replaces the cells that migrate to the wound. The corneal epithelium also functions in transferring water and ions from the stroma into the conjunctival sac.

◆ Bowman membrane: The Bowman membrane is a smooth, acellular, nonregenerating layer, located between the superficial epithelium and the stroma in the cornea. The Bowman membrane contains 60 ~70 layers of type I collagen fibers. A unique pattern of collagen fibers, regularly arranged and parallel in each layer and at right angles in successive layers, contributes to transparency of the cornea.

◆ Stroma: The stroma is the thickest layer of the cornea. It is composed of mostly type I collagen fibers that are arranged in lamellae. The collagen fibers within each lamella are arranged parallel to one another, but fiber orientation shifts in adjacent lamellae. During inflammation, lymphocytes and neutrophils are also present in the stroma. At the limbus (sclerocorneal junction) is a scleral sulcus whose inner aspect at the stroma is depressed and houses endothelium-lined spaces, known as the trabecular meshwork, that lead to the canal of Schlemm. The canal of Schlemm is the site of outflow of the aqueous humor from the anterior chamber of the eye into the venous system. (Fig. 18-3)

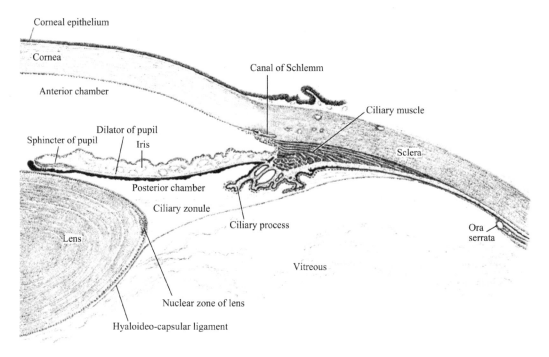

Fig. 18-3　Diagram of sclerocorneal junction

◆ Descemet membrane：Descemet membrane is a thick basement membrane interposed between the stroma and the underlying endothelium. Although this membrane is thin and homogeneous in younger persons, it becomes thicker and has cross-striations and hexagonal fiber patterns in older adults.

◆ Corneal endothelium：The corneal endothelium is a simple squamous epithelium. It is responsible for synthesis of proteins that are necessary for secreting and maintaining Descemet membrane. These cells exhibit numerous pinocytotic vesicles and the excess fluid within the stroma is resorbed by the endothelium, keeping the stroma relatively dehydrated, a factor that contributes to maintaining the refractive quality of the cornea.

ii . Sclera

The sclera is composed of type Ⅰ collagen fibers interlaced with elastic fibers. The sclera, the white of the eye, is nearly devoid of blood vessels. It is a tough fibrous connective tissue layer and gives form to the eyeball, which is maintained by intraocular pressure from the aqueous humor (located anterior to the lens) and the vitreous body (located posterior to the lens). Fibroblasts of the sclera are elongated, flat cells. Tendons of the extraocular muscles insert into the dense connective tissue surface layer of the sclera.

Ⅱ. Tunica vasculosa

The vascular middle tunic of the eye, the tunica vasculosa (uvea), is composed of three parts: iris, ciliary body and choroid.

i . Iris

The iris is a circular diaphragm and takes up one third part of the uvea and separates anterior and posterior chambers. Its free end is suspended in aqueous humor between the cornea and lens; and its root is continuous with the ciliary body. Its central adjustable aperture is the pupil, whose opening regulates the amount of light reaching the retina. Its anterior surface, which contacts the anterior chamber has a discontinuous layer of stromal cells: a mixture of fibroblasts and pigment-containing melanocytes. The abundant population of melanocytes in the epithelium and stroma of the iris not only blocks the passage of light into the eye but also imparts color to the eyes.

A double layer of pigmented cuboidal epithelium, continuous with that of the ciliary body, covers the posterior surface. The superficial layer of these cells is in contact with aqueous humor in the posterior chamber. The inner layer is made of myoepithelial cells, which form the dilator pupillae muscle. Postganglionic nerve fibers of the sympathetic nervous system stimulate the cells to contract, which causes pupil dilation. In the stroma lies the pupillae muscle, a flat ring of circumferential smooth muscle that reduces pupillary diameter by contraction. Postganglionic nerve fibers of the parasympathetic nervous system innervate it.

ii. Ciliary body

The ciliary body, the specialized anterior part of the uvea, has main functions of accommodation and production of aqueous humor. This wedge-shaped fibromuscular ring anchors and suspends the lens by zonular fibers, which allow changes in lens shape for accommodation. The inner surface of the ciliary processes is covered by a double-layered ciliary epithelium. The outer layer contains melanin and is in contact with a richly vascularized connective tissue. The inner nonpigmented epithelial layer is made of simple cuboidal to columnar cells. They secrete aqueous humor into the posterior chamber. The aqueous humor enters the anterior chamber through the pupil, and reaches the iridocorneal angle of the anterior chamber, and then drains the canal of Schlemm, which is the main exit route from the anterior chamber for aqueous humor. The canal of Schlemm is around the corneal circumference to drain into a plexus of veins.

Deep in the ciliary body is the ciliary muscle, which consists of three groups of smooth muscle cells, in radial, circular, and meridional orientations. Contraction of this muscle eases tension on zonular fibers, which allows the lens to become more convex, thereby altering its refractive power to accommodate for near vision.

iii. Choroid

The choroid, the well-vascularized, pigmented layer of the posterior wall of the eyeball, is loosely attached to the tunica fibrosa. It is composed of loose connective tissue containing numerous fibroblasts and melanocytes. Because of the abundance of small blood vessels in the inner surface of the choroid, it is responsible for providing nutrients to the retina. The choroid is separated from the retina by Bruch membrane. (Fig. 18-4)

III. Retina

The retina has two parts: the outer retinal pigment epithelium and the inner neural retina, containing three sets of modified neurons (photoreceptors, bipolar cells, and ganglion cells) that are linked in series by synapses. They are cross-linked by association neurons (amacrine and horizontal cells) and supported by neuroglial cells (Müller cells and astrocytes). (Fig. 18-4, Fig. 18-5)

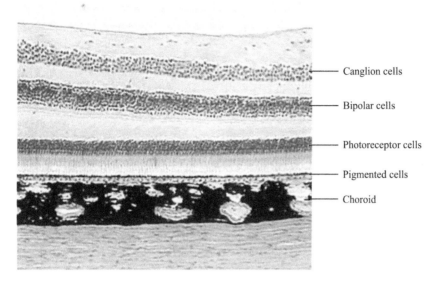

Fig. 18-4   Section of the eyeball showing the choroid and the retina

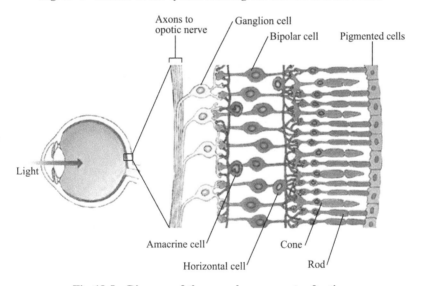

Fig. 18-5   Diagram of the neural components of retina

i . Pigmented cells

The pigmented cells are one-layered columnar to cuboidal, derived from epithelial cells and have basally-located nuclei.

The cells are attached to Bruch membrane, which is located between the choroid and the pigment cells. RER, SER and Golgi apparatus are abundant in the cytoplasm. Mitochondria are especially abundant in the cytoplasm near the numerous cell invaginations with Bruch membrane, suggesting transport in this region.

The most distinctive feature of the pigment cells is their abundance of melanin granules. The apical cytoplasm also contains residual bodies housing phagocytosed tips shed by the rods.

The pigmented cells has several functions. They absorb light after it has passed through and stimulated the photoreceptors, thus preventing reflections, which would impair focus. They continually phagocytose membranous disks shed from the tips of the rods and cones. They also play an active role in the metabolism of vitamin A, which is important for the stimulation of photoreceptors.

ii. Photoreceptor cells

The photoreceptor cells are actually the neurons, classified into two types: rods and cones. Either of the both contains inner processes and outer processes. The outer processes has outer segment and inner segment.

Outer segments consist of parallel membranous discs. Visual pigments are incorporated in disc membranes, which undergo a steady daily turnover, being progressively shed at the outer segment tips and then phagocytosed by adjacent pigmented cells. Inner segment contains organelles with abundant mitochondria. Inner processes of rods and cones synapse with bipolar cells. (Fig. 18-6)

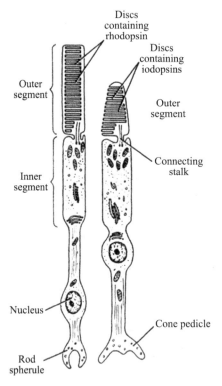

Fig. 18-6 Diagram of two types of photoreceptor cells

- ◆ Rods: Rods are narrow, cylindrical cells. In the outer segment of the rod, the membranous disk contains a specific form of the light sensitive pigments opsins, known as rhodopsin (visual purple). Rods are activated in dim light only, and are so sensitive that they can produce a signal from a single photon of light. However, they cannot mediate signals in bright light, and they cannot sense color.

- ◆ Cones: Cones are larger, shorter and conical cells. Cones are activated in bright light and produce greater visual acuity compared with rods. There are three types of cones: L cones (long wavelength), M cones (medium wavelength), and S cones (short wavelength), each containing a different variety of the photopigment opsin, known as photopsin responding to different wavelengths of light. Thus, each variety of photopsin has a maximum sensitivity to one of three colors of the spectrum: red, green, and blue.

iii. Bipolar cells

Bipolar cells are two-processed neurons and transmit impulse from rods and cones to ganglion cells via synapses. In addition, neuronal horizontal cells, amacrine cells and Muller glial cells are present in the layer of bipolar cells.

iv. Ganglion cells

Ganglion cells send axons out of the eye at the optic disc forming optic nerve.

IV. Macula Lutea

The macula lutea (yellow spot) is at rear pole of retina with central fovea in the center. The fovea only contains cones, which are thinner and longer than elsewhere, so has highest visual acuity. (Fig. 18-7)

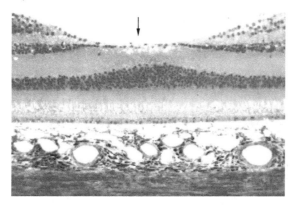

Fig. 18-7   Section of the eyeball showing the macula lutea(arrow)

V. Optic disc

The optic disc, also known as optic papilla is situated at the medial to macula lutea. It is a blind spot, because this area is the exit of nerve fibers and has no photoreceptor cells.

18.1.2   Contents of eyeball

The eyeball contains aqueous humor, lens and vitreous body.

I. Aqueous humor

The aqueous humor is the watery fluid produced by nonpigmented epithelial cells and diffusion from capillaries of ciliary body. Passes to anterior chamber via pupil, and through trabecular meshwork enters Schlemm's canal, then aqueous veins convey it to venous system. Aqueous humor functions in serving as a refracting medium, nourishing lens and cornea, and maintaining intraocular pressure. Blockage of the drainage causes glaucoma.

II. Lens

The lens is flexible, biconvex and transparent. It is suspended between iris and vitreous body by ciliary zonules.

For near vision, ciliary muscle contracts, tension on ciliary zonules lowers, lens becomes thicker and refracting power increases. For far vision reverse events occur.

With age or diseases lens becomes more rigid and opaque, this is cataract.

III. Vitreous body

Vitreous body fills cavity of eyeball behind the lens, composed of gel-like connective tissue. Its functions are providing support, nourishing and serving as the refracting medium for lights.

18.2 Ear

The ear has three parts: external, middle, and inner (labyrinth). The external ear, consisting of the auricle and external acoustic meatus, conducts sound waves from the external environment to the tympanic membrane. The middle ear (tympanic cavity) is an air-filled cavity in the petrous temporal bone that transforms sound waves into mechanical vibrations. Lined by a mucous membrane, it contains three auditory ossicles and communicates with the nasopharynx via the auditory (eustachian) tube. The inner ear has special receptors for hearing and maintenance of equilibrium. The bony labyrinth in the inner ear contains perilymph, which surrounds the endolymph-filled membranous labyrinth. (Fig. 18-8)

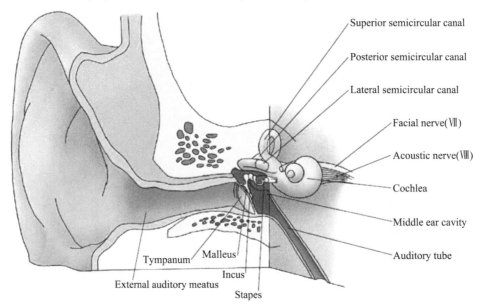

Fig. 18-8 Diagram of ear

18.2.1 Inner ear

The inner ear consists of bony labyrinth and membranous labyrinth.

I. Bony labyrinth

The bony labyrinth, composed of the semicircular canals, vestibule, and the cochlea, is a series of communicating channels hollowed out in the petrous temporal bone. (Fig. 18-9)

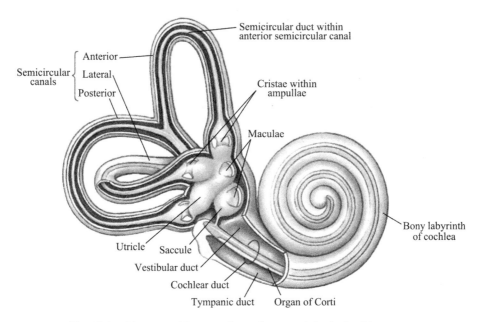

Fig. 18-9   Diagram of bony and membranous labyrinth of inner ear

ⅰ. Semicircular canals

The three semicircular canals (superior, posterior, and lateral) are oriented at 90 degrees to one another. One end of each canal is enlarged; this expanded region is called the ampulla. All three semicircular canals arise from and return to the vestibule, but one end of each of two of the canals shares an opening to the vestibule; consequently, there are only five orifices to the vestibule.

ⅱ. Vestibule

The vestibule is the central portion of the bony labyrinth located between the anteriorly placed cochlea and the posteriorly placed semicircular canals. Its lateral wall contains the oval window and the round window.

ⅲ. Cochlea

The cochlea, a spiral canal shaped like a snail shell, is embedded in temporal bone. It coils two and one-half times around a central bony column, the modiolus. From the modiolus, projects into the spiraled cochlea with a shelf of bone called the osseous spiral lamina, from which a connective membrane, tectorial membrane, is given rise to.

Ⅱ. Membranous labyrinth

The membranous labyrinth is suspended within the bony labyrinth, including three parts: semicircular ducts, utricle and saccule, and   cochlear duct. The system of ducts and chambers are composed of a thin layer of connective tissue lined with simple squamous epithelium except in the crista ampullaris, maculae and spiral organ of Corti.

ⅰ. Crista ampullaris

Suspended within the semicircular canals are the semicircular ducts. The ampullae contain the cristae ampullares, which sense angular acceleration. Each crista ampullaris is composed of a ridge whose free surface is covered by sensory epithelium consisting of hair cells and supporting cells. The supporting cells sit on the basal lamina, whereas the hair cells do not; rather, the hair cells are cradled between the supporting cells. Covering the crista ampullaris is a gelatinous mass called the cupula. The free surface of hair cells has a nonmotile kinocilium and many stereocilia. Stereocilia are embedded in the cupula. Upon angular acceleration (rotation), the endolymph within the semicircular duct deflects the cupula against the hair cells of the crista ampullaris, and give rise to an impulse, thus the circular movements of the head are sensed by crista ampullaris. (Fig. 18-10)

ii . Maculae of utricle and saccule

The vestibule houses specialized regions of the membranous labyrinth, the utricle and the saccule. Maculae of the utricle and the saccule have senses of linear acceleration and gravity. Their sensory epithelium has two types of cells: hair cells and supporting cells, all resting on a basement membrane. A macula hair cell has

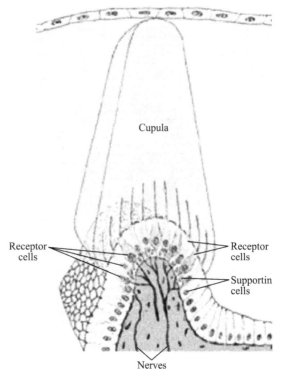

Fig. 18-10　Diagram of crista ampullaris

one kinocilium and many stereocilia that project into the gelatinous otolithic membrane. Calcium carbonate crystals make up the otoliths, which are suspended on top of the gelatinous layer. Macula hair cells are innervated at their bases by both afferent and efferent nerve fibers of the vestibular part of cranial nerve Ⅷ. (Fig. 18-11)

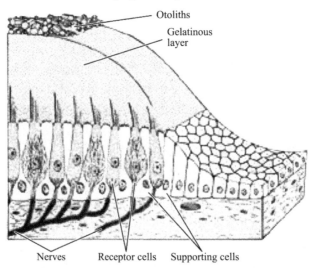

Fig. 18-11　Diagram of maculae of utricle and saccule

iii . Cochlear duct and organ of Corti

The cochlear duct is suspended within the cochlea channel, separating the latter into three compartments: scala media (cochlear duct), scala vestibuli, and scala tympani. The cochlear duct is filled with endolymph; perilymph fills the other two scalae. The scalae vestibuli and tympani communicate through the helicotrema, a small opening at the cochlear apex.

♦ Cochlear duct: The cochlear duct is a triangular space in transverse section. Its lateral border makes up the stria vascularis-a richly vascularized pseudostratified epithelium that secretes endolymph. Reissner's (vestibular) membrane, which marks the roof of the cochlear duct, delineates cochlear duct from scala vestibuli. A thicker basilar membrane forms the floor of the cochlear duct and separates it from scala tympani. Superimposed on the basilar membrane is highly specialized epithelium, organ of Corti.

♦ Organ of Corti: Organ of Corti consists of supporting cells and hair cells (Fig. 18-12).

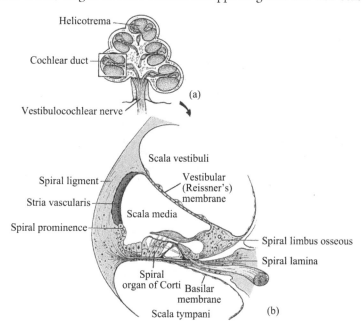

Fig. 18-12   Diagram of cochlear duct and organ of Corti

♦ Supporting cells: A single row of Inner and a single row of outer pillar cells are tall cells with wide bases and apical ends. They are attached to the basilar membrane, and each one arises from a broad base. The central portions of both inner and outer pillar cells are deflected to form the walls of the inner tunnel. A single row of inner and three rows of outer phalangeal cells are tall columnar cells that are attached to the basilar membrane. Their apical portions are cup shaped to support the basilar portions of the outer hair cells.

♦ Hair cells: Inner hair cells, a single row of cells, are supported by a single row of inner phalangeal cells. Their apical surface contains stereocilia arranged in a " − " shape. Outer hair cells, supported by outer phalangeal cells, are located near the outer limit of the organ of Corti and are arranged in rows of three or four. Their apical surface contains stereocilia arranged in a "V" shape. The basal aspects of these cells synapse with afferent fibers of the cochlear division of afferent and efferent nerve terminals of cranial nerve VIII.

18.2.2 Functions of cochlea

Sound waves collected by the external ear pass into the external auditory meatus and are received by the tympanic membrane. Because of a mechanical advantage rendered by the articulations of the three bony ossicles and the difference between the surface area of the tympanic membrane and the foot of the stapes, the mechanical energy is amplified about 20 times when it reaches the membrane of the oval window. Movements of the oval window membrane initiate pressure waves in the perilymph within the scala vestibuli. The wave is passed through the scala vestibuli, then through the helicotrema at the apex of cochlea, into the scala tympani. The wave causes the basilar membrane to vibrate. When stereocilia of hair cells touch tectorial membrane and bend, the hair cells generate an impulse that is transmitted via the afferent nerve fibers of the cochlear division of the vestibulocochlear nerve (Fig. 18-13).

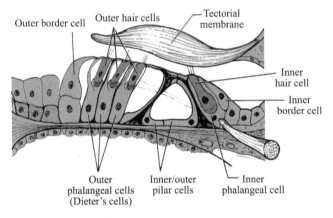

Fig. 18-13 Organ of Corti

The differences in sound frequency are distinguished because regions of the basilar membrane, which becomes longer with each turn of the cochlea, vibrate at different frequencies relative to its width. Therefore, low-frequency sounds are sensed near the apex of the cochlea, whereas high-frequency sounds are near the base.

REFERENCES

[1] William K. Ovalle, Patrick C Nahirney. Netter's Essential Histology. 2nd ed. Elsevier, 2007.

[2] Barry S Mitchell, Sandra Peel. Histology: An Illustrated Colour Text. Elsevier, 2009.

[3] Barbara Young, Phillip Woodford, Geraldine O'Dowd. Wheater's Functional Histology. 6th ed. Elsevier, 2013.

[4] Anthony L. Mescher. Junqueira's Basic Histology: Text and Atlas. 14th ed. McGraw-Hill Education, 2015.

[5] Abraham L Kierszenbaum, Laura Tres. Histology and Cell Biology: An Introduction to Pathology. 4th ed. Elsever, 2015.

[6] Michael H. Ross, Wojciech Pawlina. Histology: A Text and Atlas: With Correlated Cell and Molecular Biology. 7th ed. Lippincott Williams and Wilkins, 2015.

[7] Leslie P. Gartner. Color Atlas and Text of Histology. 7th ed. Lippincott Williams and Wilkins, 2017.